ANIMALS
PARASITIC IN MAN

Geoffrey Lapage

REVISED EDITION

DOVER PUBLICATIONS, INC.
NEW YORK

Published simultaneously in Canada by McClelland and Stewart, Ltd.
Published in the United Kingdom by Constable and Company Limited, 10 Orange
Street, London W.C.2.

This new Dover edition, first published in 1963, is a revised version of the work
first published by Penguin Books in 1957 as a volume in the Pelican Medical Series.

Library of Congress Catalog Card Number: 63-17908

Manufactured in the United States of America

Dover Publications, Inc.
180 Varick Street
New York 14, N.Y.

Contents

List of Plates

List of Text Figures

List of Text Figures

List of Text Figures

Editorial Foreword

DISEASE, the general nature of which I attempted to describe in one of my own books, may be inborn in a man. Indeed it can be handed down to him as a legacy from generation to generation. More often it is due to man succumbing to one of the many and sometimes great dangers to which we are all exposed in varying degrees in the environment in which we live. Of these one of the most important is unfortunate collision with some other form of life which shares this strange world with us. True that the larger animals have long since ceased to be any grave menace to mankind, but the smaller forms of life, which can get into or live on man's body, are now well recognized, common and widely distributed causes of disease. These latter, in so far as water-tight classification is possible, include, in ascending order of magnitude, the pathogenic viruses, the pathogenic bacteria, and the animals parasitic in or on man.

In this volume, Dr Geoffrey Lapage, who has devoted a lifetime to the study of parasitic animals and the diseases which they carry, particularly in tropical and sub-tropical countries, gives a fascinating account of the more important parasites which may affect man and cause different forms of disease in him. He explains the devious devices by which they get inside different parts of the human body; how, having got there successfully, they compete with and live at the expense of their host; how they reproduce in such a way as to ensure the survival of their race; and how many have evolved multiple and complex life cycles that have widened their distribution in organic nature. He also tells us how they cause disease in man and finally how they can be best avoided or eradicated and so the disease which they cause prevented.

This book should make an appeal to a wide circle of readers. First and foremost it will be invaluable to the medical student. For the doctor, particularly if he is likely to practise medicine in the tropics, must possess a sound working knowledge of this important subject and in these pages the medical student will find an attractive account of human parasites and parasitic disease in man to which the dry verbiage of the average text book of medicine just cannot hold a candle. In the second, it is bound to make an appeal to any layman interested in natural history. For the study of parasitology, more perhaps than that of any other branch

Editorial Foreword

of biology, illustrates and underlines how, as the result of variation and the operation of natural selection, new forms of life have evolved in the course of world history by adapting themselves to new and almost unimaginable ways of living. In the third place, it should appeal to the professional biologist who, through his study of the lives of animals in general, has become more and more interested in the life of man in particular as manifest in himself and the peculiar risks to which we may be exposed during our brief sojourn on this planet, Earth. Finally, it should prove invaluable to professional chemists engaged in the never-ending search for substances which will kill parasites in man without at the time destroying him; and to all doctors, nurses, social workers, health visitors, medical administrators, and others whose duty it is to endeavour to maintain a reasonable standard of human health in the parasite-ridden man inhabited tropical and subtropical countries of the world.

In short, Dr Lapage's book will, on the one hand, help to widen the approach of doctors, medical students, and nurses to their work, namely the prevention and treatment of disease which so besets humanity. On the other, it will enable the intelligent layman, employers of labour and all those working on the fringe of medical practice to understand the doctor's problems and to help them to work in with the medical profession. For, as I have written before, and shall never hesitate to say again and yet again, the right use of the growing power of medicine in the best interests of suffering humanity, and it is growing very fast, depends on cooperation between the four main interested parties, namely the potential patient, his doctor, the employer of labour, and society as embodied in the State.

A. E. CLARK-KENNEDY

Preface and Acknowledgements

THIS book was originally published in 1957 by Penguin Books Ltd in their Pelican Medical Series, and the gratifying sale of it in that form has encouraged the writer to revise it for publication in its present form. It attempts to provide, primarily for the reader who is not specially trained in biology or in human or veterinary medicine, a readable account of the animals that may be parasitic in man in various parts of the world. At the same time an attempt has been made to provide for the medical student, and for others who may, for various reasons, wish to learn the essential facts concerning human parasitology, accounts of the parasitic animals that cause human disease. A further aim of the book is to indicate the general principles on which the comparatively young science of parasitology is based. The last Chapter explains the battle that man is nowadays waging with animals parasitic in him and the gravity of the injury that these animals do to his health and civilization.

The line illustrations in the text have been drawn by Mr J. Walkey from sketches supplied by the author and the author is indebted to Mr Walkey for the trouble he has taken over them. The diagrams of the life histories have been specially designed for this book, but the other line illustrations are based on drawings used by the author in teaching. These latter inevitably owe much to the work of the parasitologists of many countries of the world and the author gratefully acknowledges the debt he owes to all these workers.

For the photographs the author is greatly indebted to: Dr D. Robertson, North of Scotland College of Agriculture for Plate 1 (a), and Plate 7 (b); Mr G. H. Werts, Imperial Chemical (Pharmaceuticals) Ltd for Plate 2 (b), Plate 4 (a), Plates 5 and 6, Plate 7 (a), and Plate 8; Dr H. Spencer, St Thomas's Hospital, London for Plate 4 (b); Dr Seaton, Liverpool School of Tropical Medicine and the Editor of *The Lancet* for Plate 1 (b) and Plate 2 (a); and the Director of the Wellcome Museum of Medical Science, London for Plate 4 and text figures 6 and 43.

1963   G. L.

CHAPTER ONE

What is a Parasitic Animal?

THIS book is not about bacteria, which are parasitic plants; nor about viruses, which are parasites, but are neither animals nor plants. It is about the animals that are parasitic in man, about, that is to say, such animals as the human malarial parasites, the trypanosomes that cause sleeping sickness in Africa, the mosquitoes, tsetse flies, horse flies, and other insects that either suck human blood or otherwise annoy man, and about the host of parasitic worms – a whole rogues' gallery, you may say. But are they the rogues that they seem to be? It is natural that we human beings, who live, or try to live, independent, self-supporting lives, during which we give, or try to give, an adequate return for all that we take from our world, should dislike, or even be horrified by, the parasite which lives, as our dictionaries tell us, at the expense of other living things and gives nothing in return for what it takes. Quite rightly we despise, in our human society, the person who lives in this way, the sycophant, the hanger-on, the sponger who does no work and contributes nothing to the pool of human needs, but lives on the efforts of others, or even goes further and does his fellows harm. This, in our human language, is the meaning of the word parasite, which stands, in the minds of normal men and women, for a way of life that we view with disdain, disgust, or downright condemnation.

But this view of the parasite, right though it is when it is applied to civilized man, cannot be accepted by the biologist. Biologists study, by methods that are as scientific as they can be made, the ways of life, not only of man, but of all kinds of living things, whether they are plants or animals or viruses. They neither approve nor condemn the truths that they find. They take off, so to speak, their human spectacles and try to see life as it is. If we do this, we see the parasites, not as disgusting or despicable creatures, nor even, if we can be sufficiently dispassionate, as creatures that do man, and other forms of life, a great deal of harm, but simply as creatures that use, in the fascinating maze of ways of living, a particular method of getting that basic necessity that all living things must get, namely, their food.

How do parasites get their food? By considering this we shall arrive, by a process of exclusion, at a definition of a parasite. It will not be, it cannot be, the clear-cut definition, free from all qualifications, that human thinkers so often vainly seek; for life is not static, nor fixed in process or form; it is fluid, dynamic, always subject to continuous change. It cannot, therefore, be neatly pigeon-holed and classified: we cannot put, so to speak, a pattern of compartments over living things and, labelling one for parasites, put all our parasites neatly into that. We shall find, indeed, that, although many parasites can be so separated off, there will always be many which will not fit into our pigeon-hole; these will belong to more than one of our human categories. They link the parasite to the creatures that live in other ways; and, because they do this, they often show us how the parasite has come, in the passage of time since life on the earth began, to adopt the mode of life which is its mark and character. What is this parasitic mode of life? We shall understand it best if we compare it with two other modes of life adopted by plants and animals, namely the two modes of life called symbiosis and commensalism.

Symbiosis, commensalism, and parasitism are three of the categories into which the ecologist – the biologist who studies the ways of life of living things and their relations to their environments – divides what he calls *associations* of living things, which live together for various reasons. These associations may be formed between animals only, plants only, or animals and plants. They may be, as herds of cattle, flocks of sheep, the communities of ants, bees, and wasps or the colonies formed by corals are, associations between individuals belonging to the same species; or they may be associations between individuals belonging to different species. Commensalism, symbiosis, and parasitism all belong to this latter category.

The term commensalism, which means 'eating at the same table', was originally given to associations between two or more animals belonging to different species which share each other's food. Some sea-anemones, for instance, settle on the shells of crabs and feed on scraps of food not eaten by the crabs. But nowadays some authorities extend the term commensalism to include species which derive from their association with other species, not only food, but benefits of another kind. The oxpicker bird in Africa, for instance, perches on the backs of rhinoceroses, elephants, and other African mammals, feeding upon the lice and ticks on these animals; the mammals upon which the birds perch derive from the association warning of the approach of danger, because the oxpicker, when danger approaches, reacts to it by flying away. It is said that the not uncommon sight of starlings perched on the backs of sheep in England, where they feed on the lice, keds, and ticks that live in the wool of the sheep, may serve the sheep in a similar way. Another benefit derived by some of the partners in other commensal associations is shelter from the rigours of the environment. There are, for example, prawns that find shelter by living inside sea-cucumbers and shrimps that live inside sponges. The canals inside sponges may, in fact, give shelter, and no doubt, food also, to many different kinds of animals. In the loggerhead sponge, for instance, as many as 17,128 other animals, belonging to ten different species, have been found.

The parts played by the different partners in associations of this kind are various. They vary from the association of two partners each of which provides some kind of benefit to the other, to associations in which one or more of the partners does not contribute anything to the association. The mark of these commensal associations is, however, the fact that, whether or not one or more partners contributes nothing to the association, none of the partners in the association suffers any harm. They may all benefit from it, or only one or some of them may; but none of the partners suffers any handicap or injury.

15

They are all, moreover, independent individuals, all of which are capable of leading independent lives. Physiologically, the most that any partner gets is a supply of food, which it must catch, eat, and digest for itself. There is no organic connection of the tissues of any of the partners with those of any of the other partners.

These two features of commensalism, and incidentally, of all the categories into which it is sometimes subdivided, distinguish commensalism from both symbiosis and parasitism. Symbiosis resembles commensalism in one respect. It is an association between different species of animals neither of which suffers any harm from the association. It goes, in fact, further than commensalism does. It provides, in its characteristic form, definite benefits for the partners in it. Usually there are only two partners and each derives some essential part of its food from the other. It goes further than commensalism in another characteristic way. The two partners in a symbiotic association are so closely associated with each other that their tissues are in physiological communion. You can take, for example, the sea-anemone away from the crab in which it lives in commensal association and the crab and the anemone can live apart from each other; but you cannot thus separate the two partners in a truly symbiotic association. By themselves they cannot live. They may be able, for the purposes of reproduction of their kind, to separate for a while; but their young, when they have been reproduced, must take up the symbiotic association again. The reason for this is that the association depends on a physiological association between the actual tissues of the two partners in the association. In our ponds and streams, for instance, there is a small fresh-water coelenterate, a relative of the sea anemones, called *Hydra viridis*. The green colour is due to the presence, inside its body, of a single-celled green plant called *Zoochlorella*, which produces, as green plants do, oxygen and sugar, and the *Hydra* uses these and produces waste matter containing nitrogen, which the *Zoochlorella* needs. More familiar to some readers as an example of symbiosis is the group of plants called the lichens. These are all examples of the association between two different kinds of

What is a Parasitic Animal?

plants, an alga and a fungus, which live together all their lives, providing each other with substances necessary to their lives.

These symbiotic associations, marked as they are by the intimate association between the actual tissues of the two partners, and also by the loss of the power of independent life, remind us at once of many typical instances of parasitism. In parasitism too – at least in its typical form – there is loss of the power of independent life. In many instances, but not in all, parasitism also involves a close association between the tissues of the partners in the association. The difference lies in the effects on the partners. In symbiosis both partners benefit. In parasitism only one partner, the parasite, derives benefit. The other partner, appropriately called the *host* of the parasite, gets nothing from the partnership. It gives the parasite food, and in many instances it gives the parasite other benefits, such as shelter from the effects of the environment. So accustomed, indeed, may the parasite become to living inside its host, that it cannot any longer survive in the world outside the body of the host. But the host gets nothing in return. It suffers, in fact, not only from the failure of the parasite to give it anything in return, but also from the actual injury to its body inflicted by the parasite. This injury may be done when the parasite takes its food; it may nibble off pieces of the host, or it may suck the host's blood, or it may injure it in the other ways described later in this book. The host, in response to the invasion of its body by the parasite, fights back and does all it can to minimize, or localize, or heal, the injury done to it by the parasite. Parasitism, therefore, is a one-sided partnership, a state of conflict that is in striking contrast to the harmony of the symbiotic relationship. Its hallmarks are the resistance made by the host and the injury done by the parasite.

The host's resistance, and the injury done by the parasite, may be great or small. If the injury done is sudden, or great, and the host's resistance is slight, the host may be quickly killed. This is the mark of relatively recent, unsuccessful parasitism, which has not yet had time to evolve, by a slow process of adaptation of host and parasite to each other, towards those other forms of parasitism in which the host, although it un-

17

doubtedly suffers injury, is injured so little, or fights back so successfully, that the parasite makes little or no difference to its life or health. It may be difficult, indeed, where we find host and parasite thus living together in a state of what we call *tolerance* of each other, to decide whether these are instances of parasitism, or even of symbiosis.

Parasitism, however, can always be infallibly distinguished by one fact. Parasites always injure their hosts. The harm done may be very slight; it may be visible only with the aid of a microscope; or other methods of investigation, such as serological or biochemical reactions, may be required to show that it is there: but it does exist; and it marks the dividing line between parasitism and all other forms of association between living things.

So far, however, we have considered parasitism only in relation to symbiosis and commensalism. We have established it as a particular way of getting food and can say that a parasite is an organism, whether it be a plant, a virus, or an animal, that gets its food from the bodies of other organisms which are called its *hosts*, and that, as it does this, it inflicts a degree of injury on these hosts. Is this enough to define the parasite? Does it, someone will say at once, distinguish the parasite from the predator? The tiger, it can be argued, and the microscopic carnivores that range through the green and quiet dells in our ponds and streams, these are getting their food from the bodies of other animals and these, too, harm their prey; they kill them, in fact, which is more than the parasite usually does. Extending our view beyond the animal world, we may consider the cow that crops our fields, the rabbit that does our crops so much harm, the plants indeed, that feed on insects and other prey, and decide that all these seem to fulfil our definition of the parasite. How can they be distinguished from the parasite?

The distinction has been well expressed by Elton (1935) who has said that: 'The difference between a carnivore and a parasite is simply the difference between living on capital and income . . . .' The parasite, that is to say the typical parasite, does not destroy the animals or plants on which it feeds; it

18

compromises, as Elton further points out, between getting the food it requires and not destroying this source of food. The death of its host means its own death, or at least so much less of the food it cannot do without. It does not, to put it another way, kill the goose that lays the golden eggs.

The parasite moreover, is usually smaller and weaker than its host. It is true that some predators – the weasel for example – are smaller than the animals they prey upon; but the great majority of parasites are all much smaller than their hosts. Among the parasites that are animals all, except very few, are invertebrates. Vertebrate animals are, no doubt, too bulky to be able to make a success of parasitic life and most of them are so well-equipped for a free and independent existence that they have not been led into the exploration of parasitism. Only a few of them have taken to it. Examples of parasitic vertebrates are the blood-sucking bats considered in chapter 10; and the hag-fishes, those relatives of the lampreys that do so much damage to fish. Hag-fishes bury their cylindrical heads in the bodies of their hosts and consume their tissues, often until the host-fish dies.

One other feature of parasitism needs a word or two before we try to define the parasite as precisely as we can. This is the distinction often drawn between parasites which live only on the surfaces of the bodies of their hosts and those which live inside their bodies. The former are called *external parasites* or *ectoparasites*; examples of them are the lice and fleas and the mites that cause human scabies. Contrasted with these are the *internal parasites* or *endoparasites*, which live either in the food canal of the host, which is, in effect, a portion of the exterior enclosed within the host, or in the host's blood or other tissue-fluids, or in its muscles or other organs. In order to reach these internal organs, these internal parasites pass, either through the host's mouth, which is the portal of entry most often used; or they penetrate through the host's skin; or less often, they enter the host through such natural openings on its surface as the openings that lead into the respiratory, genital, or urinary organs. They hardly ever enter the host through the vent (*anus*). In other instances, some other kind

19

of parasitic animal, such as a mosquito, horse fly, sand fly, or tick, which visits the host to suck its blood, injects the internal parsite through the skin of the host.

The distinction often drawn between the external and internal parasites is, however, mainly a topographical one. It has its uses, but it does not help us much when we are considering the effects of parasites on their hosts; for then we have to consider, among other things, the reactions to the parasite of the whole host's body when it acts as a single, integrated organism. When we consider these reactions of the host, we learn that attacks made by the parasite on the surface of the host often cause reactions in its internal organs as well, so that the distinction between external and internal parasites loses the value that it at first sight seemed to have.

There are, in addition to this distinction between internal and external parasites, other distinctions which do not affect any definition of the way of life called parasitism. There is, for instance, the distinction sometimes drawn between temporary and permanent parasites. *Temporary parasites* are such species as the mosquito and the horse fly, which visit their hosts only at times, only, in fact, when they need the blood of the host which is their food. These species are non-parasitic in every other respect, but, because they feed on their hosts, they are undoubtedly parasites. They may be contrasted with species that are sometimes called *permanent parasites*, which are parasitic throughout the whole, or the greater part, of their lives. Many temporary parasites are, as we shall see, important because, in the act of sucking blood, they convey to their hosts the causes of serious disease of the host. Such causes may be either other parasitic animals, such as the trypanosomes or the malarial parasites, or bacteria or viruses.

Some parasites, on the other hand, are parasitic only when the opportunity for parasitic life becomes available. Normally they lead non-parasitic lives. The maggots, for example, of the blowflies and the bluebottle and copperbottle flies normally develop in dead flesh or in decaying vegetable material; but, if their parents, attracted to sheep, or even to man, by the smell of pus in septic wounds or sores, or by the odours of excrement adhering to wool or hair or the skin, lay their eggs in this kind of material, the maggots may become truly parasitic on the sheep or other host and may feed on the tissues of that host and cause the formation of severe abscesses and other lesions. Anyone who has seen a sheep suffering from the disease called strike of sheep, will realise the extent of the damage that these maggots may inflict. Parasites of this kind, which can live either a parasitic or a non-parasitic life, are called *facultative parasites*. They are contrasted with *obligatory* parasites, which must be parasitic and can live in no other way.

Other categories of parasites are useful, but they need only brief explanation here. Some species of parasites are, for instance, parasitic on other parasites and these are called *hyperparasites*; their hosts are, so to speak, victims of their own mode of life. There are also the wandering or *aberrant* parasites, which are individuals of any parasitic species which stray, for various reasons, from the routes inside the host's body that are normally followed by the species to which they belong. Their departures from these routes lead them to unusual tissues or organs, in which they cannot live, so that usually they die in these situations. We have to recognize, too, certain species of parasitic animals that may be found in the bodies of hosts in which they do not normally occur. Man, for example, may occasionally be the host of species that are not usually parasitic in, or on the surface of, his body. These parasites, when they attack an unusual host, are called *occasional*, or *accidental* parasites of that host. The common liver fluke of sheep and cattle, *Fasciola hepatica*, may, for instance, become parasitic in man.

It is important to know what species are normally parasitic in each host, and also what other species may sometimes be parasitic in that host, because, unless we know this, we do not know all the sources from which the infection of a particular host, such as man, may be derived. We have to remember, too, that the excreta of a particular host, such as a human being, may contain the eggs or other phases of parasites that cannot be parasitic in that host, but may have been swallowed by the host, so that they are passing through its digestive canal. The faeces or urine of man, for example, may contain not only the eggs and other phases of parasites that cannot be parasitic in man, but even such non-parasitic organisms as the caterpillar or pupae of insects, or even adult insects that are not parasitic in any animal. There may also be seeds, imperfectly-digested remains of food, starch-grains, and other objects that may resemble parasites or phases of their life histories. To all these objects, whether they belong to parasitic or non-parasitic species, or to the food of the host, the general name *pseudoparasites* is sometimes given.

We are now in a position to say, as precisely as we can, what a parasite is. A parasite, we can say, is a living organism which establishes a physiological association with the tissues on the surface of, or inside, the body of another organism, which is usually bigger and stronger than the parasite and always belongs to a different species, the purpose of this association being primarily to provide food for the parasite; this other organism is called the host of the parasite and the host always suffers, as a result of its association with the parasite, some degree of injury and always reacts to some degree against the parasite and the injury that it suffers.

This definition is, we must admit, not entirely satisfactory. It attempts, as all other definitions of living organisms do, to confine, in a static framework, something that is slowly and continuously undergoing change. It does, however, focus attention on the parasitic animals that are the subject of this book. It gives us, however, no hint of the variety and complexity of the world of parasites, nor of the beauty of the structural and physiological adaptations that they show; nor even, on the other side of the picture, of the long history of pain, suffering, and death for which parasitic animals are responsible. Man, in this book, is the host with which we are primarily concerned; and man, like other animals, has suffered, without a doubt, from parasitic animals since the earliest days of his history. There is no part of his body, nor, indeed, any part of the bodies of the hosts of parasitic animals in general, which is not visited by some kind of parasitic animal at some

What is a Parasitic Animal?

time or other during their life histories. What kinds of animals use man as a suitable host? How do they succeed in getting into his body or on to the surface of it? And what are the lives of these parasitic animals like, what are their life histories? The next chapter will help us to begin, at any rate, to answer these questions.

CHAPTER TWO

The Kinds of Parasitic Animals

THE phrase 'kinds of animals' means, so far as this chapter is concerned, the zoological classification of the parasitic animals with which this book deals. They belong, as indeed most of the parasitic animals also do, to five only of the major groups (*Phyla*) into which the Animal Kingdom is divided. These phyla are:

1. The single-celled *Protozoa*, (figs. 1, 6, 7, 43, 49), which are distinguished from bacteria and viruses by the fact that their bodies have attained what is called the *cellular grade of organization*. Their bodies, that is to say, are cells, a cell being

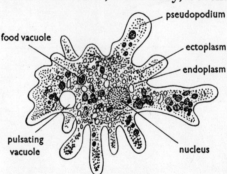

Fig. 1. *Amoeba proteus*, a common non-parasitic amoeba found in ponds and streams. An example of the single-celled Protozoa

a unit of protoplasm governed by a structure called its *nucleus*, which contains a specialized material called *chromatin*. The nucleus governs the life of the cell and the cell cannot live without it. The bodies of all the higher animals and plants are made up of cells, but the body of each of the species of Protozoa usually consists of only one cell. In the bodies of bacteria, on the other hand, the chromatin is not organized to form a definite nucleus and the bodies of viruses are, so far as we know them at present, even more primitive than this. Examples of Protozoa parasitic in man are *Entamoeba histolytica* (fig. 6), which causes human amoebic dysentery and the human malarial parasites.

2. The ringed worms or *Annelida* (fig. 2). This phylum in-

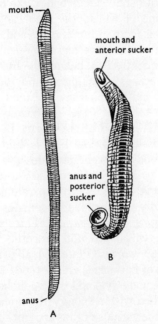

mouth

mouth and
anterior sucker

anus and
posterior
sucker

B

anus

A

Fig. 2. Two ringed, segmented worms (Annelida). A, an earthworm (*Lumbricus terrestris*); B, the medicinal leech (*Hirudo medicinalis*)

cludes the earthworms, the lugworms of our sea shores, and the leeches, a few of which are parasitic on man. The leeches are described in chapter 10.

3. The *Nemathelminthes*. This phylum includes, among other species, the Class *Nematoda* or Roundworms (Plate 3a, b,

Plate 4a) some of which are parasitic in man. Many of the
Nematoda are not parasitic; they live in the soil, in the sea,
in freshwater, in almost any situation, in fact, that provides
them with sufficient moisture; but some of them are parasitic and these may cause serious diseases of man and other
animals. Nematodes are cylindrical, smooth-skinned worms,
which do not show on the surfaces of their bodies the con-
centric rings that all the Annelida show. Frequently they
are pointed at both ends. Their bodies are built on the plan
of two tubes, one of which, the food canal, is inside the
other, which is made up of the muscles and the skin outside
these. A mouth at the anterior end opens into the food
canal, which frequently has, behind the mouth, a muscular
pharynx, which acts as a sucking pump with which the food
is sucked in; behind the pharynx the food canal runs as a
straight tube to the vent (*anus*), which is usually just in
front of the posterior end of the worm. Between the food
canal and the muscles and skin there is fluid under pressure
which gives the body form and provides a resistance against
which the muscles act. Nematodes are usually unisexual;
the sexes are, that is to say, in separate individuals, the
males being usually smaller than the females.

4. The *Platyhelminthes* or *Flatworms*. This phylum includes
the eddyworms, which are not parasitic; and the flukes
(Plate 1a) and tapeworms (Plate 1b), all of which are parasitic. The bodies of flatworms are flattened so that the back
comes near to the underside and the whole body is solid, the
interior being filled with a spongy tissue called the *parenchyma*, in which the various organs are embedded. The parasitic species (flukes and tapeworms) have hooks, or suckers,
or both, with which they hold on to their hosts. Most of the
flatworms are hermaphrodite, the male and female sexual
organs being in the same individual.

5. The *Arthropoda*. This phylum includes the Class *Crustacea*,
to which the lobsters, shrimps, crabs, woodlice, and their
numerous relatives belong; the Class *Myriapoda*, which includes the centipedes and millipedes; the Class *Insecta*, examples of which are the mosquitoes, tsetse flies, house flies,

and other insects considered later in this book; the Class *Arachnida*, to which belong the king-crabs, scorpions, spiders, ticks, and mites; and a Class called the *Onycophora*, which includes species of the genus *Peripatus*, which form a link between the Arthropoda and the Annelida.

The name Arthropoda given to this phylum refers to the fact that all the species of the phylum have jointed limbs, similar to those of a lobster or a shrimp. Originally each segment of the body of an arthropod had one pair of these jointed limbs. The limbs, have however, been modified to perform various functions. Those present on the head, for example, have been modified to form eyes, feelers (*antennae*), or mouthparts which deal with the food. Other limbs further back on the body have been modified to form walking legs, swimming organs or, in the insects, wings for flying. The bodies of arthropods are entirely enclosed in a covering composed of chitin, in which other substances, such as calcium carbonate, may be incorporated. This covering forms a skeleton placed, not inside the body, as the skeletons of vertebrate animals are, but on the outside of the body. It is therefore called the *exoskeleton*. Arthropods become, as they grow, too big for this exoskeleton and they cast it off at intervals during their growth and replace it with a new and bigger one. These periodic moults of the exoskeleton are called *ecdyses* and ecdyses are characteristic of the life histories of all arthropods. The sexes of arthropods are typically in separate individuals, but some of them show important modifications of the sexual process, such as the production of young without fertilization of the egg (*parthenogenesis*) and other modifications with which this book is not concerned. The arthropods considered in this book include a few species of Crustacea, which help to transmit tapeworms and roundworms to man, a number of species of insects, which are either temporary parasites of man or transmit other species of parasitic animals to him, and the species of Arachnida, such as the ticks and mites which are either parasites of man or transmit to him bacteria or other causes of disease. The phylum Arthropoda

27

also includes certain species of centipedes, scorpions, and spiders, which may inflict on man dangerous bites or stings.

DIRECT AND INDIRECT LIFE HISTORIES

The anatomy of all these different kinds of animals cannot be fully described in a book of this size, but succeeding chapters will give, as the mode of life of each parasitic species is described, the anatomical features that are necessary for a clear understanding of the parasitic associations that these species have established with man and their other hosts. Before we go on to consider these species, however, an important general feature of their life histories must be explained.

The term life history is given to the whole series of changes of structure and adaptation experienced by any animal, whether it is parasitic or not, between the moment when its life begins in the fertilized egg, or, among the single-celled Protozoa, the equivalent of the fertilized egg, and the time when it reaches the phase of the life history which, in its turn, produces fertilized eggs or their equivalent. This final stage is called the adult stage, although among the single-celled Protozoa it may be given different names. The life history of a butterfly, for instance, begins with the fertilized egg laid by the female butterfly, from which a young caterpillar (*larva*) hatches out. The caterpillar feeds and grows and eventually changes into a chrysalis (*pupa*). Inside the pupa the adult butterfly is formed and this lays more fertilized eggs, so that the life history begins again.

In a similar way the life histories of parasitic animals include a series of changes of structure which end with an adult stage, or, among the Protozoa, its equivalent; and it is necessary to know all these different phases of the life histories of all the different species of parasitic animals, because they are all closely associated with, and adapted to, the parasitic animal's need to establish and maintain a parasitic association with its hosts. Another reason for knowing all these phases is the fact that knowledge of them enables us to understand better how each parasitic animal gets from one host to another, how, that is to say, the host is infected; we can then devise methods of trying to prevent infection with them. Thorough knowledge of the details of each life history also enables us to devise effective means of attacking the parasitic animals. It shows us, so to speak, the weakest points in the cycle of changes that occur during the life history and we can then try to attack these points and to disrupt the cycle and make the life of the parasitic animal impossible.

In the following chapters the life histories of the species of parasitic animals considered will be described in some detail, but, before these details are considered, it is helpful to point out and emphasize a very important difference between two main types of life history that parasitic animals show. These two types of life history are called *direct* and *indirect* life histories respectively. The difference between them can best be explained by considering an example of each of them.

Direct Life Histories

The life history of the human hookworm, *Ancylostoma duodenale* (fig. 3), is an example of a direct life history. The adult male and female worms live in the small intestine of man and produce there fertilized eggs, which pass out of man in his intestinal excreta. Inside each egg a single young worm develops and this is called the *first larva*. The first larva hatches out of the egg and feeds on bacteria in the human excreta. It grows and moults its skin to become the *second larva*, which also feeds on bacteria. The second larva, when it is fully grown, moults its skin as the first larva did and thus becomes the *third larva*. The third larva, however, does not feed. It lives on reserves of food contained in its intestinal cells. It cannot develop further unless it becomes parasitic inside another host. Its function is to infect this host and, for this reason, it is called the *infective larva*. It is the only one of these earlier larval phases that is able to infect another host. In this particular instance the infective larva infects another host, that is to say, another human being, by boring its way through the skin, although it can also infect this host if it is swallowed with water or food. Once inside man, the infective larva becomes

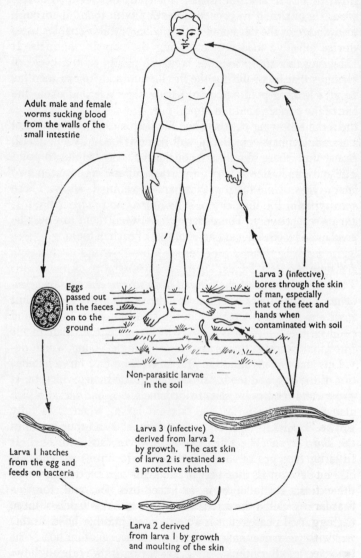

Adult male and female worms sucking blood from the walls of the small intestine

Eggs passed out in the faeces on to the ground

Larva 3 (infective) bores through the skin of man, especially that of the feet and hands when contaminated with soil

Non-parasitic larvae in the soil

Larva I hatches from the egg and feeds on bacteria

Larva 3 (infective) derived from larva 2 by growth. The cast skin of larva 2 is retained as a protective sheath

Larva 2 derived from larva I by growth and moulting of the skin

Fig. 3. The direct life history of a human hookworm

parasitic in the small intestine, where it feeds and grows and moults its skin to become the *fourth larva*. The fourth larva then grows up to become either a male or a female adult worm.

During this life history the parasitic animal is, it will be observed, parasitic only during the later phases of the life history. The earlier phases are not parasitic and the whole life history can be divided into a non-parasitic phase, consisting of the fertilized egg, and the first, second, and third larvae, and a parasitic phase, consisting of the third and fourth larval phases and the adult worms, which produce the fertilized eggs. The parasitic animal, moreover, passes, by means of its infective larva, *directly* from one host to another. It lives, so to speak, its life without any help from any other kind of animal except its hosts. In these it produces fertilized eggs, which pass out of the host and enter another host when the infective larva has been formed. Species with life histories of this type are thus the lone hands, so to speak, of the parasitic world. They find their hosts and live inside them entirely on their own; all that they need is a host in which they can produce fertilized eggs.

Indirect Life Histories

Let us now look at the life history (fig. 4) of *Fasciola hepatica*, the common liver fluke of sheep and cattle, which may, under circumstances explained in chapter 5, become parasitic in man.

The adults of this species are parasitic in the bile ducts of the livers of sheep, cattle, and other vertebrate hosts. In this situation they produce fertilized eggs, which pass out with the bile into the small intestine of the hosts and ultimately reach the exterior in the droppings of the hosts. Inside each egg a first larva called a *miracidium* develops and this hatches out of the egg. It is covered with small protoplasmic hairs (*cilia*) and with these it swims in water on the pastures on which the hosts feed. It lives thus a brief non-parasitic life. It must, however, become parasitic inside a certain species of amphibious or aquatic snail. If it does not succeed in getting into one of

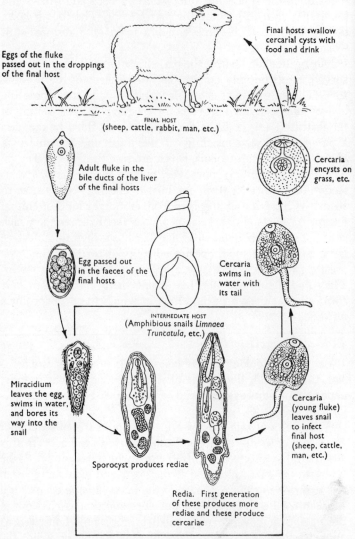

Eggs of the fluke passed out in the droppings of the final host

Final hosts swallow cercarial cysts with food and drink

FINAL HOST
(sheep, cattle, rabbit, man, etc.)

Adult fluke in the bile ducts of the liver of the final hosts

Cercaria encysts on grass, etc.

Egg passed out in the faeces of the final hosts

Cercaria swims in water with its tail

INTERMEDIATE HOST
(Amphibious snails *Limnaea Truncatula*, etc.)

Miracidium leaves the egg, swims in water, and bores its way into the snail

Sporocyst produces rediae

Cercaria (young fluke) leaves snail to infect final host (sheep, cattle, man, etc.)

Redia. First generation of these produces more rediae and these produce cercariae

Fig. 4. The indirect life history of the common liver fluke of sheep and cattle (*Fasciola hepatica*)

these snails, it quickly dies. Inside the snail it develops into a second larval phase called the *sporocyst* and inside this a third larval stage called the *redia* develops. Each sporocyst may produce many rediae. Each redia may then produce inside itself a second generation of rediae; but, whether this happens or not, each redia eventually produces inside itself a number of individuals each of which is called a *cercaria*.

The cercaria is the fourth larval phase and it is the last of the larval phases. It cannot develop further unless it succeeds in entering the body of a sheep or a cow or that of any of the other hosts in which the fertilized eggs can be produced. Its function is to infect one of these hosts. It is the only larval phase that can do this. It is therefore comparable to the infective larva of the hookworms described above. It leaves the snail, swims about for a while with the tail with which it is provided and eventually settles down on a water plant, or on grass or on some other object, and there it casts off its tail and encloses itself inside a protective membrane. Inside this membrane or *cyst* it waits until it is eaten by a sheep or cow or rabbit when these animals crop the herbage. Man may infect himself by eating watercress, windfall fruit, or some other vegetable on which cercariae may have encysted. When it is eaten by one of these hosts, the cercaria, which is, in fact, a young fluke, makes its way to the bile ducts of the liver and there it becomes, in due course, an adult hermaphrodite fluke, which lays, when it is sexually mature, fertilized eggs.

This life history thus differs from that of the hookworms in one important respect. Whereas the hookworms need only the host in which they produce fertilized eggs, the liver fluke needs, not only a host in which it can do this, but also a host in which its larval phases can develop. Unless it succeeds in finding a host (snail) in which its larval phases can develop and produce cercariae, it cannot complete its life history. It must, that is to say, be parasitic not once during a single life history, but twice and in two very different kinds of animals. The host in which its larval phases develop – in this instance the snail – is called the *larval* or *intermediate host* and the host in which the fertilized eggs are produced – in this instance a sheep or a cow or a rabbit or a human being – is called the *final* or *definitive host*. It follows that the parasite cannot pass directly from one host in which it produces fertilized eggs to another host in which it can do this; it can only pass indirectly from one to another of these hosts, namely, by way of the intermediate host in which its larval phases must develop. For this reason its life history is said to be indirect.

The distinction between the final and the intermediate host is important both to the parasitic animal and to man, who wishes to prevent infection of himself and other animals with the parasitic animal. It is important to the parasitic animal because it forces this animal to be parasitic in two different kinds of animals, one the final host in which its fertilized eggs are produced and another, the intermediate host, in which its larval phases must develop. The distinction between the final and the intermediate host is important from the point of view of the control of parasitic infections, because infections of the final host can only come from larval phases of the parasitic animal produced inside the body of the intermediate host and infections of the intermediate host can only come from the products of sexual reproduction, which must occur inside the body of the final host. It follows that, when man is the final host of any species of parasitic animal with an indirect life history, he cannot infect himself with phases of this species present inside his own body, as he can when the life history is direct; he can be infected only by larval phases of the parasitic animal coming from the intermediate host; and, if he can avoid these, he can avoid the infection altogether. The same principle applies when man is the intermediate host. He can then be infected, not by phases of the parasitic animal present in his own body, but only by the products of its sexual reproduction, which must occur inside the body of the final host. Control of infections with parasitic animals with indirect life histories usually, therefore, involves the protection of man from either the intermediate or the final hosts from which the infections may come.

The species described in chapters 5, 6, 7, and 8 all have indirect life histories. The species described in chapter 7, however, introduce another complication. They are dependent not on one intermediate host only, but on two successive intermediate hosts. Their larval phases, that is to say, develop only to a certain stage in the first of these successive intermediate hosts and must complete their development in the second intermediate hosts. Only after successful development in the second intermediate hosts are they able to produce the infective larva which is able to infect the final host in which the adult phases live and produce fertilized eggs.

The distinction between the final and the intermediate host just described must not be confused with two other distinctions which are important from the point of view of the control of infections with parasitic animals. In the first place, intermediate hosts must be distinguished from what are called *transport hosts*. An intermediate host is, as has just been explained, a host in which the larval phases of a parasitic animal must develop before they can pass on to the final host. The eggs or larvae of a parasitic animal may, however, pass into animals which merely carry them about and disseminate them elsewhere. In these animals which give them transport the eggs or larvae cannot develop; they are merely passengers and the animals that thus carry them about are called transport hosts. Transport hosts are important because they may carry about the infective eggs or larvae of species of parasitic animals which may have either direct or indirect life histories. The infective larvae of the gapeworm of poultry, *Syngamus trachea*, for instance, which has a direct life history, may be carried about inside earthworms, and poultry may infect themselves by eating the worms. Among species which have indirect life histories which may have transport hosts, so that they must use intermediate hosts and may also use transport hosts, is the broad tapeworm of man, *Diphyllobothrium latum*, described in chapter 7, the infective larva (plerocercoid larva) of which may, when fish eat each other, pass from the fish in which they develop and which are the second intermediate hosts, into other fish, in which they cannot develop further, so that these latter fish are transport hosts.

The second distinction which is important is the distinction

35 1275814

between intermediate and final hosts and what may be called *alternative hosts*. Most species of parasitic animals, whether their life histories are direct or indirect, can live in more than one host and these various hosts in which the parasitic animal can live are its alternative hosts. Among species with direct life histories, for example, many of the roundworms that cause inflammation of the food canals of sheep and cattle can live equally successfully in deer, antelope, and other ruminant animals. Similarly species with indirect life histories may have several intermediate and several final hosts in which they can live. The common liver fluke of sheep and cattle, *Fasciola hepatica*, for instance, can use, in different parts of the world, a number of different species of snails as its intermediate hosts and its adult phase can live in sheep, cattle, horses, pigs, rabbits, man, and other animals.

This ability to live, however, in several alternative hosts is not by any means a characteristic of all species of parasitic animals. Some of the species with direct life histories have relatively few alternative hosts. *Entamoeba histolytica*, for instance, the amoeba which causes amoebic dysentery of man, can live in man and the dog, but in practically no other animals. And some species with direct life histories are restricted to only one species of host. *Enterobius vermicularis*, for example, is confined to man and cannot use any other animals as its hosts. In the same way some species with indirect life histories are confined to certain intermediate and final hosts only. Some can use few species of animals, or only one kind, as intermediate hosts and many kinds of animals as final hosts; some can use several kinds of animals as intermediate hosts and only a few kinds as final hosts; and some, such as the human malarial parasites, can use only one kind of animal, namely man, as the intermediate host and only one kind of animal, namely mosquitoes belonging to the genus *Anopheles*, as the final host. These latter species have therefore become very rigidly restricted to a narrow range of parasitic activity.

It will thus be evident that all species of parasitic animals have, whether their life histories are direct or indirect, one or more hosts with which they are normally associated. These are called their *normal*, *usual*, or *principal hosts*. Each parasitic animal is, however, usually able to live in certain other hosts in addition to these, though these are hosts in which it is not so successful as it is in its normal hosts. These other hosts are called its *abnormal*, *unusual*, or *occasional* hosts.

In any event each parasitic animal is limited to a certain range of hosts. It is, that is to say, *specific* to these hosts and cannot live in others. This *host-specificity* is an important feature of parasitism and it will be necessary to refer to it throughout this book. It will be evident, for instance, that if a particular host, such as man, is one of the usual hosts of a certain species of parasitic animal, it is necessary, if we wish to prevent the spread of this parasitic species, to know what its other usual hosts are, and also what its unusual or occasional hosts are, because all these hosts may be sources from which the parasitic animal may spread. These other hosts are reservoirs of the infection and they are called *reservoir hosts*.

Often, but not always, we find that parasitic animals do less harm to their usual hosts than to their unusual or occasional ones. They have, in the course of their history, become relatively well adapted to life in association with their normal hosts. This adaptation may, in fact, go so far that the parasitic animal does relatively little harm to its normal hosts. These hosts, to put it the other way round, tolerate the parasitic animal. Frequently they tolerate it because they have developed some form of resistance (immunity) to it. In some instances the toleration has developed to such an extent that the parasitic animal does so little harm that the host's health is hardly affected at all. It may, indeed, then be difficult to distinguish this kind of parasitism from commensalism. In other instances commensal associations may, for reasons that we do not understand, become parasitic ones, because one of the partners in them begins to do harm to the other. The amoeba (*Entamoeba histolytica*), for example, which causes human amoebic dysentery, lives as a harmless commensal in the large intestines of many human beings; but it may, for reasons that

37

we do not yet know, abandon its commensal life and invade the walls of the large intestine and do damage there that causes amoebic dysentery. Its life history and habits are further described in chapter *3*.

CHAPTER THREE
The Lone Hands

IN this chapter and the next one, species which have direct life histories will be described. All of them are parasitic in man and two of the aims of this chapter are to show some of the routes by which parasitic animals may enter the human body or the bodies of other animals, and to illustrate important principles of the host-parasite relationship. It will be possible also to indicate some of the ways in which the species described may injure man. The species to be considered first are the human hookworms which cause so much illness in Africa, Asia, parts of North and South America, and also in parts of Europe. They used to attack man in England in the tin mines of Cornwall and they were, until they were eradicated, common also in the people working in mines in France and Germany.

THE HUMAN HOOKWORMS
Plate 3b

These worms belong to the group of parasitic worms called the Roundworms (*Nematoda*), but the name roundworm is not a good one, because the bodies of roundworms are cylindrical. They are 'round' only in the sense that the cross-section of them has an approximately circular outline. Like all roundworms, the human hookworms have a smooth skin (*cuticle*), which is not marked by rings that are visible to the unaided eye, as the skins of earthworms, leeches, and their relatives (*Annelida*) are. The cuticle of roundworms is semi-transparent, so that the straight food canal and the coils of the male or female sexual organs may be visible through the skin. Because the hookworms suck blood, they are often coloured reddish by blood in their food canals. The blood is sucked in through a bell-shaped structure round the mouth at the anterior end. Inside the mouth there are teeth or cutting plates, with which the worm abrades the soft lining of the small intestine of the host. It may suck in a plug of this lining (fig. 5) and bite

39

off portions of it with its teeth, or it may penetrate into the wall of the small intestine till it reaches a small blood vessel.

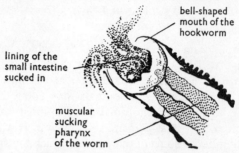

Fig. 5. A human hookworm sucking in and nibbling
the lining of the small intestine of man

It then injects into the host substances, called *anticoagulins*, which delay or prevent the clotting of the blood, so that a plentiful supply of blood is available. The blood thus sucked from the host is passed quickly through the food canal of the hookworm and out again at the anus, which is near the posterior end of the worm's body, but not, as it is in the earthworms and their relatives (*Annelida*), at its posterior tip. The amount of blood thus removed from the host is further discussed in chapter 12. It may be considerable and the loss of it causes the anaemia which is a prominent symptom of the disease caused by hookworms. We do not know what use the hookworms make of the blood that they remove. Because they usually suck blood from small arteries rather than from small veins, it seems probable that they use the respiratory pigment (*haemoglobin*) in the blood for their own respiration and that the blood is therefore not sought as food, but to enable the worms to breathe.

Hookworms belong to the family of roundworms called the Ancylostomatidae. The following species of this family may be parasitic in the small intestine of man:

Ancylostoma duodenale

This is a greyish-white species, but it is reddish when it has been sucking blood. The males are 8 to 11 mm. ($\frac{3}{10}$ to $\frac{4}{10}$ inch) and the females 10 to 13 mm. ($\frac{4}{10}$ to $\frac{1}{2}$ inch) long. The males

40

are thus smaller than the females, as the males of roundworms usually are. *Ancylostoma duodenale* is sometimes called the Old World hookworm. It attacks man in Southern Europe from Italy to Bulgaria, in North Africa, in northern and parts of southern India and also in north China, Japan, Malaya, and Indonesia. In the Americas it occurs in the southern United States and the West Indies and, in South America, Venezuela, Brazil, Peru, and Chile. It has been suggested that it was brought to America by Chinese labourers and by Chinese people who settled in America.

Ancylostoma braziliense

This species is rather smaller than *Ancylostoma duodenale*, the males being 7·8 to 8·5 mm. and the females 9 to 10·5 mm. long. Its normal hosts are dogs and cats, in which it occurs in the small intestine. In man it is occasionally found in the south-eastern United States, along the coasts of the Gulf of Mexico, in north and central South America and also in India, Ceylon, Burma, and Indonesia.

Ancylostoma ceylanicum

This species is only occasionally found in man. It occurs in Asia and South America. Normally it is parasitic in the dog. It is about the size of *Ancylostoma duodenale*.

Necator americanus

The name of this important species means 'American Murderer' and it refers to the fact that this is the species of hookworm most often found in man in the United States. It is therefore sometimes called the American or New World hookworm. It occurs in tropical and sub-tropical parts of the world and is responsible in these areas for 90 per cent of hookworm infections. As its name implies, it is the predominant species in the Americas, where it occurs in the southern United States and central and northern South America, but it is also found in Central and South Africa, central and eastern India, China, parts of Japan, Burma, and Indonesia down to the north-east coast of Australia. It is smaller than species of the genus

Ancylostoma, the males being 5 to 9 mm. ($\frac{1}{5}$ to $\frac{2}{5}$ inch) and the females 9 to 11 mm. ($\frac{2}{5}$ to nearly $\frac{1}{2}$ inch) long. It has been suggested that it was taken to America in the bodies of Africans who were imported to that country as slaves and also perhaps in the bodies of other people who immigrated to America.

It is difficult to estimate the number of people in the world who are infected with *Necator americanus* and species of the genus *Ancylostoma*, because the geographical distribution of the species of these two genera varies; but Stoll (1947) estimated that 457 million people in the world were, at the time when he made his investigations, infected by one species or another of these genera of hookworms.

The Life History of Hookworms

The life histories of all the species of human hookworms are similar. They have already been outlined in chapter 2, but they may be given in rather more detail here. The adult male and female worms live in the small intestine of man, where they suck blood. They produce fertilized eggs, which are passed out in the excreta of the host. Inside the eggs a young worm, called the *first larva*, develops and this hatches out of the egg and feeds on bacteria in the human excreta, until it has grown too big for its skin. It then moults its skin and becomes the *second larva*, which also feeds on bacteria and moults its skin to become the *third larva*. The third larva is formed in about a week, or less, after the first larva left the egg. It also moults its skin, but this moulted skin is kept on this larva as a loose sheath which protects the third larva inside it to some extent from the injurious effects of its environment. Because this third larva is thus enclosed inside the cast skin of the second larva, it cannot feed and must rely on reserves of food stored up in its intestinal cells.

The three larval phases just described, which live in human excreta or in soil on to which these excreta have been deposited, are all non-parasitic and the formation of the third larva marks the end of this non-parasitic phase of the life history. The function of the third larva is to infect a new host, either by entering this host through its mouth, or by penetrating through its skin. It is the only one of the three non-parasitic larval phases that can do this and, if the host swallows the first or second larvae, these are killed in the host's food canal. For this reason the third larva is called the *infective larva*. It is an active creature, about 0·5 mm. ($\frac{1}{50}$ inch) long. Although it can infect the host through the mouth, it usually infects the host by penetrating the skin. The larvae of some other species of parasitic animals can also infect their hosts by penetrating the skin and they are called *skin-penetrating larvae*. Another example of them among the parasitic animals that infect man is the larva of Bancroft's filarial worm described in chapter 5.

Normally men, or dogs, or cats, or any of the other hosts of hookworms, become infected by third infective larvae present in soil over which the host walks with uncovered ankles or feet, or in soil which is handled by the host. These larvae are present in the soil because the soil has been contaminated with the excreta of the hosts, which contain the eggs from which the third larvae develop. Man can therefore be infected only by soil contaminated by his own excreta and, if contamination of the soil by human excreta could be avoided, man would not be infected with hookworms.

The third infective larvae are relatively easily killed by being dried, so that they survive best in warm, moist soil. For this reason they, and in consequence the adult worms also, are most prevalent in the soils of the warmer countries of the world. If they survive elsewhere, they are found in soil in sheltered and humid places. They can, for instance, survive in certain places in the soils of Europe, especially in southern Europe, especially in the warmer and more humid places. The soils of mines and other underground places provide them with a suitable environment and they were a scourge of the labourers who made the St Gotthard Tunnel in Switzerland. Some of these labourers, when they returned home to work in the mines of Germany, Holland, Belgium, and England, brought the hookworms with them, so that the infection was a scourge of miners in these countries, until it was eradicated by the hygienic and other preventive measures outlined in chapter

12. It is still, however, necessary to keep a watch lest the infection return again.

When the host exposes its skin to the soil containing the third infective larvae, these larvae bore their way through the skin. Often they enter the softer skin between the toes, or through the skin of the ankles, or, when the soil gets on to the hands, through the skin of the hands or wrists. As they bore into the skin they cause intense itching and also inflammation, the signs of which are reddening of the skin and some swelling under it. A rash of small papules often develops and these become small vesicles. All this is the expression of the host's reaction against these invaders of its body and the skin-eruption caused is called *ground itch*. If the vesicles become infected with bacteria, as they may do if the infected person scratches them to allay the itching, unpleasant sores may develop.

A similar eruption in the skin of man may be caused by the larvae of certain strains of *Ancylostoma braziliense*. The normal hosts of this species are dogs and cats, but the larvae of certain strains of it may penetrate into the skin of man. The larvae of these strains only rarely develop in man into the adult hookworms, but they can penetrate into human skin and, when they do this, they may live for a time in the skin and move about in it, causing as they do so, a skin-eruption similar to ground-itch, which is called *creeping eruption*, or *cutaneous larva migrans*, because the eruption follows the migration of the larvae in the skin. Cutaneous larva migrans may also be caused by the larvae of several other species which are normally not parasitic in man. These larvae, when they get into the skin of man, cannot grow up into adults and sooner or later they die in human skin and their remains are absorbed. Among the species whose larvae cause skin irritation in this way are the hookworms of dogs and cattle and the bot-flies of horses. Cutaneous larva migrans must be clearly distinguished from *visceral larva migrans*, described on p. 62.

A similar eruption of the skin may be caused by the larvae of another roundworm, *Gnathostoma spinigerum*, the adults of which live in tunnels that they cause in the stomachs of cats and their wild relatives and also in the stomachs of dogs. The eggs of this species, passed out in the excreta of these hosts, hatch in fresh water and liberate a first larva that is swallowed by the fresh-water crustaceans, *Cyclops* (figs. 19, 30), inside which this larva becomes a second larva. When the *Cyclops* is eaten by frogs, fishes, or snakes, the third larva develops inside these animals and the cats and dogs infect themselves by eating the frogs, fishes, and snakes. Man may infect himself with the third larvae by eating fish containing them and, if he does this, the larvae may wander into the skin and cause the eruption just mentioned. The larvae, however, never, so far as we know, become fully mature gnathostomas, but immature specimens have been found in abscesses or in tunnels in human skin and it is possible that this species is learning how to become fully mature in man.

Returning now to the third larvae of the human hookworms, we find that, when they are in the human skin, they find their way into the blood in the veins of the skin and are carried by them to the right-hand side of the heart, from which the blood is pumped to the lungs, where it takes up oxygen. The hookworm larvae thus reach the lungs and here they break out of the small blood vessels (capillaries) into the small air-sacs of the lung itself, which are full of air. From the air-sacs they wriggle up the breathing tubes (*bronchi*) to the windpipe (*trachea*), which opens into the back of the mouth. As they go they develop into fourth larvae. From the back of the mouth they are swallowed into the stomach and thus reach the small intestine, inside which they become adult male and female worms.

This life history illustrates certain basic principles of parasitic life. First, it is divided into two distinct phases, a parasitic and a non-parasitic phase. The eggs and the three larval phases that succeed the eggs are not parasitic. The fourth larva and the adult male and female worms are parasitic, the two phases being linked by the third larva, which is nonparasitic for the first part of its life and parasitic for the second part. The third larva thus lives in both the parasitic and the non-parasitic worlds. It has to be able to live both outside and inside the host. The third larva is, in fact, the phase of the whole life history on which the survival of this parasite depends. Its job is the vital one of establishing the parasite's association with the host. Because it infects the host, it is called the *infective phase* of the life history. No other phase of the life history can do this. If the eggs are swallowed by the host, they will not hatch inside it and, if they did, the first larvae emerging from them could not live in the host's food canal. Nor could the second larvae survive inside the host. And the fourth larvae and the adult worms, which, are parasitic, could not survive long enough outside the host to infect it from the outside. Only the third larvae can begin the life of the parasite inside its host's food canal.

A second feature of this life history is the fact that it is the older phases of the life history – in this instance the fourth larvae and the adult worms – that are parasitic, the younger phases being non-parasitic. We shall see, later on, that some parasitic animals, such as the warble flies of cattle and the relatives of these flies that may be parasitic in man, reverse this plan; their younger phases only are parasitic, the pupae and adult flies being non-parasitic.

A third feature of the life history just described is important from the point of view of the spread of infection with parasitic animals. The infective phases are *active* creatures. They are therefore able to do a little towards the solution of the problem of getting into a host. They can, for instance, put themselves into situations in which they are likely to be swallowed by the host, or to have opportunities to penetrate through its skin. Further, their ability to infect the host by penetrating through its skin gives the species to which they belong an advantage over parasitic animals whose infective phases cannot do this. It enables them to enter the host at virtually any point on its external surface and it absolves them from the dependence on the food habits of the host which governs the lives of species which can infect the host only through its mouth.

To make this point clear, let us now look at the life histories of some species that are entirely dependent on entry into the host through its mouth. These are species whose infective

46

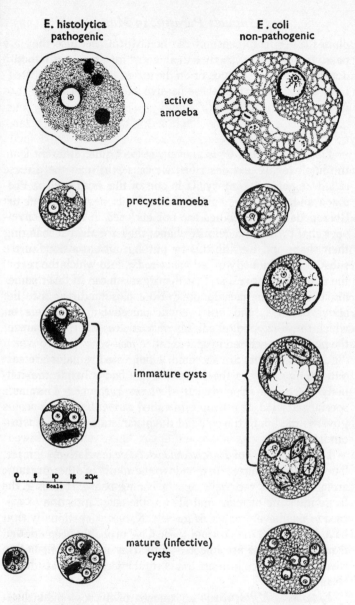

Fig. 6. The human dysentery amoeba (*Entamoeba histolytica*) and the harmless, commensal *Entamoeba coli* and their cysts

47

phases differ from those of the hookworms because they are passive, not active, so that their entry into the host's mouth depends either on chance or on the actions of a host which neglects to make sure that these passive infective phases have not got into its food or drink.

Entamoeba histolytica

This species (fig. 6) is in every respect quite different from the hookworms just described. It causes in man the disease called amoebic dysentery. It is one of the single-celled Protozoa and it belongs to the class of this phylum called the Rhizopoda, whose bodies are not enclosed in definite envelopes that preserve a definite shape; they are always changing their shape and they do this by putting out extensions of the substance of the body called *pseudopodia*, into which the rest of the body then moves, so that the organism can in this manner move along. The pseudopodia also enclose and take into the body, bacteria, and other small unicellular organisms on which the Rhizopoda feed. These particles, when they are in the body, are enclosed in spaces called *food-vacuoles*, into which digestive ferments are secreted. Undigested remains are cast out at any point on the surface of the body. Inside the cell-body there is a structure called the *nucleus*, which contains a specialized kind of protoplasm called *chromatin*. The nucleus governs the life of the cell and the organism cannot live without it.

The life history of *Entamoeba histolytica* is relatively simple. The phase of it that corresponds to the adults of other parasitic animals is called the *trophozoite*, a feeding-phase. It lives in the large intestine of man; and also in the large intestine of macacque monkeys (genus *Macacus*). Natural infections with it have been found in dogs and these have probably been derived from man. If cats are infected with it by man, it will live in them, especially in kittens; but natural infections of cats do not occur.

Entamoeba histolytica is an amoeba of microscopic size. It measures 10 to 40 (average 20 to 30) micra in diameter, one micron being one thousandth of a millimetre or about $\frac{1}{25000}$

inch. Within the variations of the size of *Entamoeba histolytica* just given, however, individuals of different sizes form what are called *biological races* of this amoeba, the individuals of which maintain more or less a constant race-size throughout their life histories.

Entamoeba histolytica is an active amoeba, and, like many other species of the genus *Amoeba*, it shows a division of its cytoplasm into an inner more granular protoplasm, called the *endoplasm* and an outer layer of clearer, non-granular protoplasm, called the *ectoplasm*. The pseudopodia formed by *Entamoeba histolytica* are quite characteristic of it. They usually consist of clear ectoplasm only and they are formed at any point on the surface of the amoeba quite suddenly, as if the ectoplasm had exploded out at the point at which they are formed. Less often the amoeba puts out a single pseudopodium in one direction only and moves in his direction at a considerable rate, so that its movement recalls the mode of progression of a slug.

In a great many of the people who become infected with it, *Entamoeba histolytica* lives as a harmless commensal in the large intestine. It feeds there on bacteria and other food material that the large intestine contains. It is only under certain circumstances that it becomes parasitic and causes disease. We do not yet understand why it thus changes its mode of life, but, when it does so, it attaches itself to the lining of the large intestine and secretes a ferment (a *cytolysin*), which destroys the cells lining the intestine, so that the amoeba is able to invade the tissues of the intestinal wall. The amoebae penetrate in this manner into the walls of the large intestine and spread along them laterally, causing the formation of the ulcers that are characteristic of amoebic dysentery. *Entamoeba histolytica* is now damaging its host and is therefore a parasite. Because it can live harmlessly in its host as well, it is a *facultative parasite*.

The life history of *Entamoeba histolytica* is a simple one. The feeding stage (*trophozoite*) that feeds on the intestinal contents or the tissues of the host, multiplies its numbers by the simple process of dividing into two amoebae. The nucleus first divides and then the cytoplasm separates into two por-

49

tions, each of which takes one of the products of the division of the original nucleus. The two amoebae thus formed then follow independent lives. This process of simple division into two is called *binary fission*; it is a method of multiplication of the number of individuals of the species that many Protozoa use. The trypanosomes, for instance, described in chapter 9, multiply in this way. Some other Protozoa multiply by the more productive method of division of the parent cell, not into two parts, but into several parts. Thus the human malarial parasites multiply inside the red cells of the blood by this method of *multiple division*, which is called *schizogony* (see chapter 8).

Binary fission increases the number of individuals present in any particular host, but it does not provide for the necessary transference of the amoeba from one host to another. The only way out of the host is by way of the excreta and these go out into the world outside the host, in which the feeding phase of the amoeba cannot live. It must therefore provide some means of survival in this outer world. This it does by forming a protected phase of itself which is called a *cyst* (fig. 6). Before it forms a cyst the amoeba divides to form smaller amoebae called *precystic forms*, and these cast out all food material except reserve food supplies. These latter take the form of *glycogen*, which is present in a vacuole in the cytoplasm; and refractile rods with rounded ends called *chromatoid bodies*. Each precystic amoeba then secretes around itself a protective *cyst-wall*. The cysts thus formed are spherical and they are 5 to 20 micra in diameter, according to the size of the race of the amoeba that formed them. Each has at first a single nucleus, which has the structural characteristics of the nucleus of the feeding stage that formed the cyst. Inside each cyst the single nucleus then divides to form 4 nuclei. The cyst is then able to infect another human being, the quadrinucleate cyst being the infective phase. The formation of four nuclei in the cyst happens before the cyst passes out of man. Cysts containing only one or two nuclei may, however, be found in human excreta, but these usually do not develop further than this, so that they cannot infect a new host.

No further changes occur in the quadrinucleate cyst until it is swallowed by another human being. The cyst then passes unchanged down the food canal as far as the small intestine, where the proteolytic ferment trypsin, present in this part of the food canal, dissolves away the wall of the cyst and thus liberates the quadrinucleate amoeba from the cyst. It may be liberated as soon as $4\frac{1}{2}$ hours after the cyst has been swallowed. The nuclei in this quadrinucleate amoeba then divide to form eight nuclei and the cytoplasm then divides to form eight small amoebae each of which has only one nucleus. The original single amoeba that formed the cyst thus gives rise in the new host to eight smaller descendants.

Entamoeba histolytica is, when it is living a harmless commensal life in the large intestine of man, only one of many harmless organisms that live in this part of the intestine. All organisms that live in this manner in any animal, or in the excreta of animals after they have been passed out of the animal, are called *coprozoic* species, species, that is to say, that live in, and on, the *kopros*, or dung. The parasitologist must be able to recognize all these coprozoic species in every host that he has to examine and he must know which of them are parasitic and therefore capable of causing disease and which are harmless. He must know, for instance, not only *Entamoeba histolytica*, which is capable of causing disease, but also the harmless amoebae and the harmless flagellated Protozoa and other organisms that may be found in the large intestine of man. Among the amoebae that may be confused with *Entamoeba histolytica* is its relative *Entamoeba coli* (fig. 6), which is a very common commensal in the large intestine of man. It is larger than *Entamoeba histolytica*, measuring 10 to 50 micra in diameter, although races of it, different in size and similar to the races of *Entamoeba histolytica*, are found. Its cytoplasm is denser than that of *Entamoeba histolytica* and it contains numerous food vacuoles, in which bacteria, yeasts, and other food materials are being digested. It shows relatively little differentiation between ectoplasm and endoplasm and its movements are very sluggish and amount, as a rule, to little more than changes of shape. Its nucleus, also differs from that of *Entamoeba histolytica*. The nuclei of both these species (fig.

51

6) are small vesicles enclosed in a membrane called the *nuclear membrane* and each nucleus has a central grain of chromatin called the *karyosome*, with other grains of chromatin arranged along the inner side of the nuclear membrane. In the nucleus of *Entamoeba histolytica* the karyosome is always central in the nucleus, while in the nucleus of *Entamoeba coli* it is not only larger, but it is also not quite in the centre. The grains of chromatin on the inner side of the nuclear membrane of *Entamoeba histolytica* are fine grains and they look like a row of tiny beads of equal size. In the nucleus of *Entamoeba coli* the corresponding grains are coarser and they form a dense ring.

The life history of *Entamoeba coli* resembles that of *Entamoeba histolytica*, but inside the cyst, the original single nucleus divides to form eight, not four, nuclei and cysts of *Entamoeba coli* can always be distinguished by this fact, as well as by the fact that these nuclei are visible in the living cyst, while those in the cysts of *Entamoeba histolytica* cannot be seen without the use of either stains that colour them or reagents that kill them and so render them visible. The nuclei in the cysts of *Entamoeba coli* are, moreover, structurally similar to those of the feeding phase and may therefore be distinguished from those which resemble those of the feeding stage of this species. There is in the cyst of *Entamoeba coli* a glycogen vacuole similar to that seen in the cyst of *Entamoeba histolytica*, but it has usually disappeared from the cyst of *Entamoeba coli* by the time that four nuclei have been formed; in the cysts of *Entamoeba histolytica*, on the other hand, this vacuole may persist to this stage. Finally, chromatoid bodies are not so often seen in the cysts of *Entamoeba coli* as they are in those of *Entamoeba histolytica*. When they do occur they have the shape of filaments or splinters with pointed ends, or of sheaves of these.

The subsequent life history of *Entamoeba coli* resembles that of *Entamoeba histolytica*, except that the cyst already contains the 8 nuclei which will become the nuclei of the 8 descendants. When, therefore, the 8-nucleate amoeba escapes from the cyst in the new host, further division of its nuclei does not occur and it divides at once to form 8 small amoebae.

Balantidium coli

Before the life history of *Entamoeba histolytica* is compared with that of other parasitic animals, it is useful here to describe briefly another parasitic protozoon which may be found in the large intestine of man and may cause a form of dysentery called balantidial dysentery. This species is *Balantidium coli* (fig. 7). It has the doubtful distinction of being the largest protozoan parasite of man. It is also very commonly found in the large intestine of the pig and may be found in some monkeys and in the rat. It belongs to the Class of Protozoa called the Ciliophora and to the Order of this Class called the Ciliata. The names Ciliophora and Ciliata refer to the fact that the locomotor organs of species belonging to this Class and Order are typically short protoplasmic processes called *cilia*, which are not very different from flagella, but they are shorter. The numerous cilia all over the bodies of these organisms bend together in unison and propel the protozoon along in the fluids

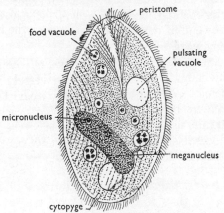

Fig. 7. The ciliate protozoon, *Balantidium coli*,
the cause of balantidial dysentery

in which it lives. Cilia in action look to the human eye much as a cornfield looks when a breeze passes over it and makes the cornstalks bend and then return to their erect position. The bodies of members of the Order Ciliata, to which *Balantidium* belongs, are typically covered with rows of these cilia.

Ciliophora all have, not one, but two, nuclei. One is large and is called the *meganucleus*; it governs the general life of the cell. In *Balantidium coli* it has the shape of a sausage or kidney (fig. 7). The other nucleus is small and is called the *micronucleus* (fig. 7). It becomes active only when the sexual processes of the organism begin. The body of *Balantidium coli* is oval and measures 50 to 80 micra long and 40 to 60 micra broad. At its anterior end there is a groove, called the *peristome*, provided with longer cilia. This groove leads to the mouth (*cytostome*), from which a gullet (*cytopharynx*) leads to the endoplasm of the cell. The food consists of particles of the contents of the large intestine of the host and also bacteria; and, when this species becomes parasitic, the red blood cells of the host and fragments of the lining of the walls of the host's large intestine are also eaten. The long cilia of the peristome waft the food into the mouth and cytopharynx and the food, when it reaches the endoplasm, is enclosed in food vacuoles like those of *Entamoeba histolytica*. Food that is not digested is passed out at an opening called the *cytopyge*, which is situated at the posterior end of the cell-body of the organism. There are two *pulsating vacuoles*.

During its life inside the host *Balantidium coli* multiplies its numbers by dividing, as all Ciliata do, transversely into two, this process being started by division of the two nuclei. When conditions inside the host become unfavourable, or when other factors not yet fully understood impel it to leave the host, the organism encloses itself inside a protective envelope, much as *Entamoeba histolytica* does, and becomes a *cyst* (fig. 8). The

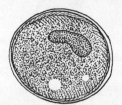

Fig. 8. Cyst of *Balantidium coli*

cyst is spherical or ovoid and has a diameter of 50 to 60 micra. The cysts are passed out of the host and may live for several weeks in the world outside the host, especially if they are not dried; but drying rapidly kills them. When they are swallowed by man, the cysts set free the individual within and the life history starts again.

Balantidium coli is found in the human intestine in most parts of the world, but, although it is common in pigs, it is not often found in man. In Britain, for instance, it is common in pigs, but is comparatively rarely found in man. Usually it is found in people who have been working with pigs. In pigs it does not cause disease, and in man it may be, as *Entamoeba histolytica* also may be, a harmless commensal that causes, so long as it lives in the contents only of the large intestine, no symptoms of disease. But if, as sometimes happens, it invades the walls of the large intestine and feeds on the tissues and red blood cells there, it becomes parasitic and causes the formation of ulcers and a serious form of dysentery, called balantidial dysentery, results.

These two life histories, those of *Entamoeba histolytica* and *Balantidium coli*, have one feature in common that differentiates them from the life histories of the hookworms described above. The two Protozoa multiply their numbers while they are inside the host, while the roundworms do not. The entamoeba, in fact, also multiplies its numbers after it has left its host and produces thus not the single infective phase derived from each of the roundworm's eggs, but eight amoebulae, each of which can start a new life history in the host. These eight descendants are, moreover, not sexually differentiated. Whereas it is necessary for the parasitic roundworms, if its species is to survive, that both male and female individuals should succeed in surviving in the host, the dysentery amoeba has not yet acquired the handicaps, and advantages, of sexuality. We shall see, later on, that some kind of parasitic animals, such as the tapeworms and flukes, are neither asexual nor unisexual, but hermaphrodite and can, like the dysentery amoeba, multiply, during their life histories, the number of individuals that may develop into the adult parasitic phase.

If we now look at the life histories of the dysentery amoeba and the parasitic roundworms discussed above from the host's point of view rather than from that of the parasite, we find that, although the parasite has gained some advantage by multiplying both its numbers inside the host and the number of individuals that can infect the host, this advantage is, to some extent, counterbalanced by the fact that its infective phase, the cyst, is a passive object, which is unable to move and is therefore dependent on the chance that it may be picked up by the host. It can, moreover, infect the host only through the host's mouth. In this respect the dysentery amoeba is in a less favourable position than parasitic animals whose infective phases are, as those of the hookworms are, active and can either place themselves in situations in which they are likely to enter the host through its mouth or can enter the host by some other route, such as through the skin, as the infective larvae of the hookworms do.

The use by parasitic animals of passive infective phases, however, has not, whatever its disadvantages may be, seriously handicapped them in the struggle for life. It is used by many species of parasitic animals and almost certainly it was one of the earliest methods of entering a host to be evolved. It is certainly the method used by most of the animals parasitic in man, the majority of which enter his body through the mouth. Usually entry through the mouth involves the production of a phase of the life history, such as an egg enclosed in a tough shell, or a cyst with a resistant wall, which can resist the injurious physical influences, such as cold, frost, drying, or the direct rays of the sun, which would, without the protection of a resistant envelope, kill the infective phase. In the next chapter we shall consider the life histories of one species which provides the contents of its egg and the infective larva that develops inside the egg with a tough, resistant envelope of this kind. This, however, is not the only method of protecting the infective phase that is used by parasitic animals which infect their hosts through the mouth. The human threadworm, also considered in the next chapter, shows us another method by which the risks of life outside the host may be reduced; and the third species considered in the next chapter shows us how the risks of life outside the host may be eliminated altogether.

CHAPTER FOUR

The Lone Hands
(CONTINUED)

=====

Life cycle

The Large Roundworm of Man (Ascaris lumbricoides)

THIS species (Plate 4a) is parasitic in the small intestine of man. Like the human threadworms, it is parasitic only in man. In the small intestine of the pig, however, there is a species which is so like the *Ascaris lumbricoides* found in man that the two can be distinguished only by means of rows of small teeth on the lips of the species found in the pig. Usually therefore these two worms are regarded as strains of the species, one of which can be parasitic only in man, while the other is parasitic only in the pig. The human species can, with difficulty, be made to live in pigs that have been kept on diets deficient in vitamin A, but biologists who have tried to infect themselves with the species found in the pig have found that, although the larvae of the pig-strain will live and develop to a certain stage in the body of man and also in the bodies of guinea-pigs and other animals, they cannot become adult in man or these other animals. The human strain of *Ascaris lumbricoides* is thus, like the human threadworm, a parasite restricted to a single host.

Ascaris lumbricoides is one of the largest of the roundworms, the male being 15 to 30 cm. (6 to 12 inches) long and 2 to 4 mm. ($\frac{1}{12}$ to $\frac{1}{6}$ inch) in diameter. The smaller males are more slender and their posterior ends are curved round towards the rest of the body. The worms of both sexes are, when they are freshly taken from the intestine of a man or pig, white or pink and they have a thick, smooth cuticle which glistens when it is wet, so that it has somewhat the appearance of wet porcelain.

This species occurs in man all over the world. It is, and

probably always has been, one of the commonest parasites of man. As Chandler (1955) says, it has 'clung to man successfully throughout the stone, copper, and iron ages.' Stoll (1947) estimated that, at the time when he made his investigations, *Ascaris lumbricoides* was present in about 644 million people in the world. It is, however, rare in Britain, although it is common enough on the Continent of Europe. Its effects on man may be, if the worms are not numerous, comparatively slight, but they may cause indigestion, discomfort and pains in the abdomen, diarrhoea, and inflammation of the bowel. When the worms are numerous, these symptoms are intensified and may simulate those of gastric and duodenal ulcer and other abdominal diseases. *Ascaris lumbricoides* has, moreover, a tendency to wander from its home in the small intestine and the worms may then enter other organs in which they may cause serious trouble. They may, for instance, enter the bile duct that brings the bile from the liver to the small intestine and may block this up, so that jaundice and other troubles result; or they may get into the appendix and cause appendicitis; and they may get into extraordinary situations, such as the ear or the genito-urinary tract. Masses of the worms in the intestine may get entangled to form a mass that may block up the intestine, so that intestinal obstruction results (Plate 4a)

The life history of *Ascaris lumbricoides* is shown in fig. 9. It may be compared with the life history of the hookworms shown in fig. 3. The adult female *Ascaris* produces, in the small intestine of man, fertilized eggs which are passed out in the excreta of the host. These eggs (fig. 9) are provided with remarkably resistant shells, which enable them to survive in the world outside the host. Inside them, when conditions in the environment of the eggs are suitable, a first larva develops, but this does not hatch out of the egg as the first larva of the hookworm does. It remains inside the egg and grows there, feeding on reserves of food that it contains, until it has cast its skin and become a second larva. Development of the larval phases inside the egg then ceases until the egg is swallowed by a new host. The egg of *Ascaris* is, in other words, the infective phase of its life history. It is, for this reason, called the

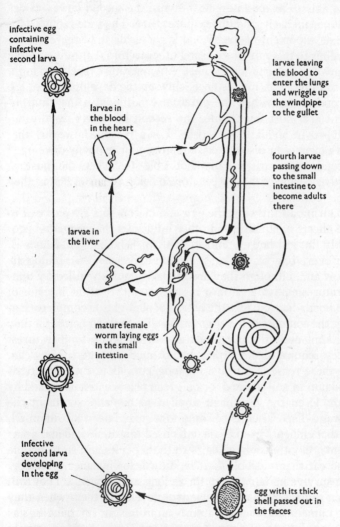

infective egg
containing
infective
second larva

larvae in
the blood
in the heart

larvae in
the liver

mature female
worm laying eggs
in the small
intestine

Infective
second larva
developing
in the egg

larvae leaving
the blood to
enter the lungs
and wriggle up
the windpipe
to the gullet

fourth larvae
passing down
to the small
intestine to
become adults
there

egg with its thick
shell passed out in
the faeces

Fig. 9. Life history of the large roundworm *Ascaris lumbricoides*

infective egg. It is not, however, infective – it is not, that is to say, able to infect a new host – until the second larva has developed inside it; and this requires time. The time required for the development of the second larva inside the egg varies according to the temperature and other factors that influence the egg while it is outside the host. A temperature that is too high, or too low, will, for instance, slow up the development of the second larva. When the external conditions in the environment are most favourable, the second larva has usually developed in about three weeks. For a reason, however, that has never been discovered, eggs containing newly-developed second larva are usually not able to infect the host, a further period of three weeks or so being required before they can.

During all this time the egg and its contents are exposed to the effects of climatic and other influences that may, and probably do, kill large numbers of them. The egg of *Ascaris* is, however, one of the most resistant objects that biologists know and, although they are relatively quickly killed by temperatures equivalent to, or higher than, that of the interior of the host's body, or by the action of sunlight or complete drying, the contents of the egg remain alive for long periods if they are kept even slightly moist and at moderate temperatures. They require also a little, but not much, oxygen. They can, for these reasons, survive for long periods in such situations as damp in soil or sand, or on green plants eaten uncooked by man. Even the treatment applied to human excreta in the sewage-disposal units of some town may fail to kill them all, so that effluents from these units used to water salad and other plants may transfer the eggs to these plants and so to people who eat them uncooked. It is known, for instance, that they can survive in damp earth for as long as five years. They will even remain alive and larvae will develop in them when they are immersed in such apparently unpromising surroundings as weak solutions of formalin; and antiseptic substances normally used for cleansing and sterilization have little or no effect upon them unless they are used in solutions so strong that they damage also the surfaces and substances to which they are applied. The larva of *Ascaris* is thus very efficiently protected during its life outside the host.

When the egg containing the second infective larva is swallowed by man, its shell is weakened by the digestive juices in the small intestine and the second larva hatches out. It at once bores into the wall of the small intestine and finds its way into the small veins in the intestinal wall. The main function of these veins in the wall of the small intestine is to collect food materials from this part of the intestine and to take it to the liver. The general direction of the blood stream is therefore towards the liver, and the larvae of *Ascaris*, when they enter the blood, are carried by it to the liver with the food. Some of them, however, make their way directly through the tissues to the same organ.

In the liver the larvae pause for a while and may, as they move about in this organ, damage it. But they do not stay long in the liver. All the blood that leaves the liver goes to the right-hand side of the heart and it takes the larvae with it. From the right-hand side of the heart the blood goes to the lungs to be aerated and the larvae of *Ascaris* are swept on by it to the lungs. Some of them may be carried on by the blood through the lungs and back to the heart and thus, in the arterial blood, to the rest of the body; but these eventually die without growing up to the adult stage. Most of the larvae stay in the lungs and moult their skins twice there, thus reaching the fourth larval stage. They then break out of the blood vessels into the air-sacs of the lung, causing, as they do this, bleeding into the air-sacs. The result of this damage may be that the host reacts against the larvae, the reaction taking the form of a condition rather like pneumonia. If the larvae are numerous in the lung, the host may then suffer shortness of breath, cough, and other symptoms that resemble those of inflammation of the lungs. The damage done, however, is relatively soon repaired and the lungs become, if they do not become infected with bacteria, healthy again. Long before this happens, however, the larvae, which are now fourth larvae, have wriggled up the air-passages to the windpipe and, reaching the back of the mouth, have been swallowed down into the stomach. Passing through this they reach the small intestine from which their journey began, and there they grow and moult their skins once more to become the immature adult male and female worms. In two to three months they become sexually mature and begin to produce the fertilized eggs with which the life history began.

Their adult lives last, however, only a year or less. This exceeds the life of the adult female human threadworm, which is numbered in days; but it is, in comparison with the longevity of some species of roundworms, a relatively short life. The adult of the human hookworm, *Ancylostoma duodenale*, for example, may live, according to different observers, for 7 to 16 years and *Necator americanus* may live for 5 to 17 years. These estimates of the longevity of roundworms parasitic in man may be compared with those given for the longevity of the tapeworms and blood flukes described in chapters 5 and 6.

A. lumbricoides has many relatives which are parasitic in many kinds of animals. They all have, in general, life histories similar to the one just described. Some of them appear to be harmless to their hosts, but others, including those found in some of our domesticated animals, such as cattle and poultry, may cause diseases of these hosts which are important to man because they may affect the health of the animals concerned and thus may affect man's food supplies. Also important are the species of *Ascaris* which are common in dogs and cats, especially in puppies and kittens. Recently it has been found that the infective eggs of these ascarids parasitic in puppies and kittens, may be swallowed by man, especially by children playing with these pets and the larvae derived from these eggs may then migrate in the human body and cause the disease called *visceral larva migrans*, which should be clearly distinguished from *cutaneous larva migrans* mentioned on p. 44.

Comparison of the life history of *Ascaris lumbricoides* with that of the hookworms shows differences that are important when we are thinking of trying to prevent the infection of man with *Ascaris*. In the first place the infective larva of *Ascaris* cannot, as the infective larva of a hookworm can, infect man by boring its way through human skin. It is restricted to entry into man through his mouth. The infective larva is the second larva and this is enclosed within the egg. Because the egg is a passive phase, the infective larva of *Ascaris* cannot place itself in a position favourable to its entry into the host. It must wait until the egg is swallowed by the new host. Infection of man therefore always occurs by chance. Each egg, moreover, produces, as each egg of the hookworm also does, only one adult worm; and this single adult must be either a male or a female worm. The multiplication of the number of infective phases shown by *Entamoeba histolytica* and more strikingly by the flukes and tapeworms described in chapters 5, 6, and 7, does not occur during the life histories of either *Ascaris* or the hookworms. These worms therefore depend, for the continuation of their species, on the entry into the same host of sufficient larvae to provide both males and females which can produce a further generation of fertilized eggs.

The difficulties facing *Ascaris lumbricoides* are therefore considerable. To them must be added the fact that this species is restricted to one host, namely man. Although its larvae, if they get into other animals, can live in these other animals for a while, and can migrate through their livers and even to their lungs, they cannot grow to maturity, so that all the infective eggs that may be swallowed by animals other than man are useless to the species and must be written off, together with the countless eggs that are killed by frost, heat, sunlight, and other physical agencies, as losses to the species that cannot be replaced. This is, no doubt, the normal experience of many, if not all living things. A common form of response to it is the production of large numbers of eggs or other reproductive phases; and *Ascaris lumbricoides* certainly responds in this way. The numbers of eggs it produces are phenomenal. It has been estimated that a single female worm may contain as many as 27 million eggs and that each female may produce 200,000 eggs a day. It has been calculated that, if each male and female of *Ascaris lumbricoides* that mate together produce 200,000 eggs a day, the mass of eggs produced by them in a year would weigh 5 grams (about $\frac{1}{4}$ oz.). In China, American observers found that some 335 million people were infected with *Ascaris* and estimated that the weight of eggs produced in a year by the worms inside these people would be 18,000 tons. These figures give an idea of the success of this species when conditions are favourable to its infection of the host; they also show what a plague of man this particular parasitic worm can be.

Also prevalent in human beings, especially in children, and, in some parts of the world, even more commonly found, is the next species to be considered, the human threadworm, *Enterobius vermicularis*, which also infects its host through the mouth by means of an infective egg. The egg of this species is not, however, well protected from the effects of the world outside the host and this species uses interesting methods of overcoming the disadvantage of having an infective phase that is relatively easily killed.

The Human Threadworm (Enterobius vermicularis)

This species (Plate 3a), which is also called the pinworm or seatworm, is, like the hookworm, a roundworm and is therefore unisexual. It belongs to the Order Oxyuroidea of the Class Nematoda. The adults of the species of this Order are small or of medium size, the males being usually much smaller than the females. The adults of both sexes live in the intestines of vertebrate hosts. They produce fertilized eggs which pass out of the host in its faeces. The eggs are usually flattened on one side.

The males of *Enterobius vermicularis* are 2 to 5 mm. (about $\frac{1}{12}$ to $\frac{1}{5}$ inch) long, but they are rarely seen. The females, however, may be found in human faeces, especially in those of children. They are whitish, small, rather spindle-shaped worms, which measure 8 to 13 mm. ($\frac{3}{10}$ to $\frac{1}{2}$ inch) long. They have elongated tails and they are often, for this reason, called pinworms. They are also called seatworms, presumably because they may be found in human faeces or even adhering to the anal region or on soiled linen in this region.

Usually these worms, when they are mature, live in the blind sac of the large intestine called the caecum, or in the colon or vermiform appendix near to which this blind sac opens; but they may also travel up the food canal to the small intestine or stomach or even higher than this. Normally, however, after the male has fertilized the female, the female, full of fertilized eggs, travels down the large intestine to the anus and, arriving there, moves out of the host through the anus and lays her eggs on the warm, moist skin of the peri-anal region. The eggs are laid in clusters or streaks and the female may travel some distance away from the anus, so that eggs may be found, not only on the buttocks, but also else-where on the skin of this part of the host's body. Usually, when she has laid the eggs, the female dies. Her movements around the anal region cause the itching which is so well-known a symptom of infection with these worms.

The eggs each contain, when they are laid, the first larva and this larva is able to infect a new host. It can do this im-mediately after the egg is laid by the female worm, so that the period of life in the outside world required by both *Ascaris lumbricoides* and the hookworms for the development of their infective phases has been eliminated by the threadworm and the risks of this period of the life history have been reduced to a corresponding degree. The eggs of the threadworm are not, on the other hand, so well protected as those of *Ascaris lum-bricoides* are, nor are they so resistant to external influences as the eggs of the hookworms are. Their shells are thin and are correspondingly less resistant to cold, drying, and other physi-cal factors that affect them outside the host. Perhaps to com-pensate for this, they are covered with a sticky material and their stickiness enables them to adhere to the skin of the part of the human body on which they are laid, namely, the region around the anus. This part of the body is, moreover, usually warm and moist, especially at night, when the female worm lays the eggs, and warmth and moisture further the survival of the eggs or larvae of all kinds of parasitic animals. The stickiness of the eggs is also correlated with the fact that the female worm, when she comes out through the anus to lay her eggs, irritates the skin of the perianal region and causes itch-ing, which the host seeks to allay by scratching the skin with the fingers. The eggs of the threadworm then readily stick to the fingers, or get under the finger nails, especially if these are long and badly-kept, and it is not then difficult for the host to convey the eggs on the fingers to the mouth, from which the larvae inside the eggs reach the food canal in which they develop into adult worms again.

Human beings, especially children and adults whose habits are for various reasons not cleanly, often infect themselves in this manner with eggs derived from themselves. This method of infection is called *auto-infection*. The fingers contaminated by the eggs may, however, transfer the eggs to pieces of furniture, door-handles, the balustrades of stairs, books, paper-money, and other objects handled both by the infected person and by uninfected people. People who are not infected may therefore get the eggs on to their fingers when they handle these infected objects and may in this manner become infected themselves. Transference of the infection in this manner from an infected to an uninfected person is called *cross-infection*. It is a common mode of infection among the individuals in families and helps to explain why it is that, when one member of a family becomes infected, other members of that family are usually found to be infected also. It is a common method also by which individuals in communities, such as factories, schools, military organizations, or mental institutions may infect one another with this species of worm.

The eggs of the threadworm may also be distributed through the air and may be inhaled with air and swallowed. This may happen, for instance, when beds used by infected persons are being 'made'. When the bedclothes are being shaken out, the eggs may get into the air and may be breathed in by the people who are making the beds. The air and dust in schoolrooms and other places in which people congregate, and the air and dust in lavatories in these and other places, may also contain numerous eggs.

A further method of infection with this species of worm is called *retrofection*. It was discovered by the extensive researches of the Dutch doctor, Professor Swellengrebel. He found that, in spite of the most elaborate precautions taken to prevent the entry of infective eggs through his mouth, infection nevertheless occurred. He was able to prove that it then occurred by the hatching of eggs laid on the perianal skin near to the anal opening and the liberation there of larvae which then entered the body through the anus and travelled up the bowel to the large intestine where they matured. This entry of these larvae 'through the back-door', so to speak, is one of the very few instances known of the infection of a host by a parasitic animal that enters the host through its anal opening to the exterior.

Infection of a new host by the methods just described depends, of course, on the survival of the larvae inside the eggs. These larvae can survive outside the host for periods varying according to the temperature and humidity from three days to several weeks. Moisture and moderate warmth prolong the lives of the larvae; drying, and especially drying combined with cold or heat, and also the effects of direct sunlight, kill the larvae relatively soon. On the moist, warm skin of the host, or on its underclothes or night clothes, or in the shelter of its bed, the larvae find the best conditions for their lives. Those that are dispersed from the host into moist, warm situations will also survive well. But in the air, or in the dust, where drying will operate, the larvae will more quickly die. It has been estimated, for instance, that only 10 per cent or so of the eggs collected from dust contain larvae able to infect a host. For the normal process of infection, however, the transference of eggs from the favourable environment of the host's skin to the mouth of the same host, or to the mouth of a close associate of this host, such as another member of the family, this parasite is adapted so well that it is not surprising that it is one of the commonest parasites of man. Stoll (1947) has, in fact, calculated that some 209 million human beings in the world were infected with this species at the time (1947) when he conducted his investigations of the incidence in man of various species of parasitic worms.

After the infective egg has reached the mouth of the host, it passes unchanged down to the small intestine and there the digestive juices soften the egg-shell and liberate the first larva within. This larva then feeds and grows and moults its skin twice before growing up into an adult male or female worm. The immature worms may live for a while in the small intestine before they proceed to the large intestine in which they mature. The whole life history, measured from the ingestion of the egg to the appearance of the adult worms, takes from 4 to 7 weeks. In individuals who maintain their infection by transferring eggs from their own perianal regions to their own mouths, the female worms will therefore appear at the anus and cause irritation there at intervals of about the same time. This explains why individual hosts may suffer recurrence, about every 3 to 7 weeks, of attacks of the itching caused by the female worms when they emerge to lay their eggs.

Reviewing this life history, we find first that man is the only host in which this species can live. It cannot live in other animals, so that man can be infected only by infective eggs derived from other human beings. This seems at first sight to simplify the problem of avoiding infection, but in practice it is usually found that the threadworm is so well adapted to its mode of life that it is very difficult to prevent infection with it. It has, so to speak, countered the drawbacks of being restricted to a single species of host by becoming so well adapted to this host that it is one of the most successful parasitic animals that we know.

Second, we find that this species, like *Ascaris lumbricoides*, infects its host by means of a passive, not an active, infective phase. It is therefore dependent upon chance and on its survival outside the host; but chance is, in this instance, aided by the stickiness of the eggs, which readily adhere to the fingers of the host and to objects that are conveyed by the host's hands to the mouth; and on the air inhaled by the host in which the larvae may survive for a while inside the eggs. Survival outside the host is, however, relatively short. It is a matter of days or a few weeks. Transference into the mouth of the host must therefore occur relatively soon after the egg has been laid. This species cannot, that is to say, risk having to wait in the dangerous world outside the host while its infective phase develops. The female worms counter this risk, first, by keeping the eggs inside the protection of their bodies until they are laid, secondly, by laying them in a situation in which they are likely to be kept warm and moist, and thirdly by producing eggs

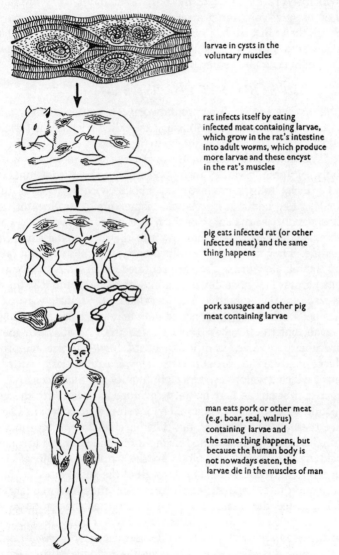

larvae in cysts in the
voluntary muscles

rat infects itself by eating
infected meat containing larvae,
which grow in the rat's intestine
into adult worms, which produce
more larvae and these encyst
in the rat's muscles

pig eats infected rat (or other
infected meat) and the same
thing happens

pork sausages and other pig
meat containing larvae

man eats pork or other meat
(e.g. boar, seal, walrus)
containing larvae and
the same thing happens, but
because the human body is
not nowadays eaten, the
larvae die in the muscles of man

Fig. 10. Life history of the trichina worm, *Trichinella spiralis*

which are ready to infect the host immediately they are laid. Let us now consider a species that has gone a step further even than this. It has solved the problem of the risks encountered in the world outside the host by the simple process of eliminating altogether the need to enter this world.

The Trichina Worm (*Trichinella spiralis*)

This species is also a roundworm. It causes in man and many other animals a serious disease called trichiniasis (trichinosis). Its life history is shown in fig. 10.

The adult male and female worms are small, the males being only 1·5 mm. (about $\frac{1}{16}$ inch) and the females 3 to 4 mm. ($\frac{1}{8}$ to $\frac{1}{6}$ inch) long, that is to say about twice as long as the males. The adults are parasitic in the small intestines of the hosts and there the union of the males and females occurs. The females, however, then burrow into the wall of the small intestine. They are full of fertilized eggs, but these are not laid by the female worm. They are retained in her uterus (womb) until a first larva has developed in each of them and it is these larvae, not the eggs, that are liberated by the female worm. It has been estimated that each female may produce about 1500 larvae, but the number produced and the rate at which they are liberated varies in different hosts. Fewer larvae are produced, and larvae are set free at a slower rate in hosts, such as man, which develop resistance (immunity) to this species.

The first larvae may be fully developed a week after the infection of the host, so that their development is rapid. They are then about 0·1 mm. long. They are set free in the spaces filled with lymph and blood in the intestinal wall and are carried by the lymph and blood to the right-hand side of the heart. The lymph vessels in the wall of the small intestine are collecting fatty products of digestion and they lead to a larger tube, called the *thoracic duct*, which empties the lymph in it into the large vein that collects venous blood from the left side of the head and neck and from the left arm (*left superior vena cava*) and this vein leads to the right-hand side of the heart. Larvae of *Trichinella* that enter the intestinal lymph spaces thus reach the right-hand side of the heart by this route.

Others enter the blood spaces in the intestinal wall and are carried, as the larvae of *Ascaris lumbricoides* are, to the liver and from there to the right-hand side of the heart.

Thus all the larvae set free in the intestinal wall reach the heart, and from this they pass with the venous blood to the lungs, but, unlike the larvae of the hookworms and those of *Ascaris lumbricoides*, they do not develop further in the lungs, nor do they travel by way of the air-passages to the food canal. They pass through the lungs and into the arterial blood and by this they are distributed all over the body of the host. Many of them doubtless die in various organs of the host. Those, however, that find themselves in the muscles that are under the control of the will (voluntary muscles) undergo further development. They penetrate into the fibres of which these muscles are composed where they feed on substances brought to them by the host's blood and grow until they are about 1 mm. ($\frac{1}{25}$ inch) long. They thus increase their length to about ten times the length of the larva that leaves the egg. Completing their growth they curl into the spiral form shown in Plate 4b and are then recognizable as male and female larvae. They are now able to infect a new host and this stage is reached in a minimum of sixteen days.

The presence of these larvae inside the muscle-fibres causes inflammation, one result of which is the formation, around each of the larvae, of a cyst-wall which shuts it off from the rest of the muscle. It has been estimated that about 1500 encysted larvae may thus arise from each of the adult female worms. Inside these cysts the larvae have no option but to wait until the muscle is eaten by another suitable host. When this happens and when the meat in which they lie helpless is digested by the host, the larvae emerge from the cysts and grow up, in the small intestine of the new host, into adult male and female worms. The adult males and females do not live long; they die about three months after the host has been infected.

This species thus relies, for its transference to another host, on the carnivorous habits of its hosts. It is not found in hosts that never eat meat. It can, nevertheless, live in some herbivorous animals, such as rodents, sheep, cattle, and horses, if it is experimentally put into the bodies of these. It is difficult, however, to get it to live in birds; and it cannot live in cold-blooded animals. It is normally parasitic in many carnivorous and omnivorous animals, all of which are mammals. Usual hosts are pigs, bears, dogs, foxes, cats, and rats and man. It has also been found even in the Arctic regions in Eskimos, polar bears, dogs, and even in white whales and seal on which the Eskimos and their dogs feed. Bear and whale meat may, therefore, be sources of human infection in these areas. Stoll (1947) estimated that, at the time when he made his investigations, about twenty-eight million people in the world were infected with *Trichinella spiralis*. From man, however, this parasite can nowadays only rarely get to other hosts. Man does not nowadays eat man and is not often eaten by other animals. In the muscles of man, therefore, the larvae usually die. They may live in human muscle sometimes for remarkably long periods of time, but eighteen months or so after the cysts have been formed around them the walls of these cysts begin to calcify and after some years the whole cyst, including the dead larva inside it, becomes calcified. Man is therefore, for this species, a blind alley from which it cannot, except in exceptional circumstances, escape.

Man is usually infected with *Trichinella spiralis* by eating the flesh of pigs that have been infected by eating rats and other infected hosts. This happens usually when pig-meat is eaten raw by man, or when the pig-meat has not been cooked sufficiently to kill the larvae in it. This question is further discussed in chapter 12.

The effects of *Trichinella spiralis* on man are to cause, while the worms are alive in the small intestine, diarrhoea and other symptoms of derangement of this part of the food canal. Later, when the larvae are being carried all over the body, severe pain, resembling the pain of 'rheumatism', is experienced. This is followed by stiffness of the muscles in which the larvae have settled down. There is often swelling and puffiness of the eyelids and face, stiffness of the jaws and an unexplained, but characteristic, appearance of black lines on the finger nails. The symptoms of infection may, however, simulate those of

72

many other diseases. Commonly they resemble those of influenza. The diagnosis therefore may be difficult. Serological tests may assist, but the only certain method of diagnosis is to remove a small portion of one of the voluntary muscles, such as a small piece of the muscle (deltoid) that caps the shoulder joint, and to examine this with a microscope. The larvae, if they are present, will then be seen.

Reviewing this life history, we can say that:

(a) This species is adapted to live inside many hosts.

(b) It relies for its transference from host to host on the use by one host of another host as prey. Its infective phase, the larva in the muscle-cyst, must be eaten by another host or it will die. For this reason this species is in nature confined to hosts that are carnivorous or omnivorous and mostly to warm-blooded mammalian hosts.

(c) It never enters the world outside the host and could not survive in this world if it did.

(d) It therefore has no need to protect its eggs or larvae from injurious influences outside the host.

Perhaps, as a consequence of this, or perhaps to increase its chances of success even inside the host, it has developed the device of viviparity. Its females, that is to say, lay, not eggs, but active larvae, which are, during their development, protected inside the body of the female worm. Considerable numbers of these larvae are produced. The life history is thus protected from the world outside the host throughout its whole course. The parasitic animal must, however, encounter and counteract the reactions of the host against it and the rapidity of its development inside the muscles of one host and in the food canal of the next one is doubtless correlated with this. We shall learn in chapter 8 that the human malarial parasites, which have indirect life histories, are also examples of parasitic animals which never enter the world outside the host and could not survive in this world if they entered it.

CHAPTER FIVE

Animals Twice Parasitic in One Life

THE species of parasitic animals now to be considered are all species with indirect life histories. They may, like the species with direct life histories already discussed, have many hosts, or only a few; they may pass, as the hookworms do, their fertilized eggs out of the host, so that there is a period of non-parasitic life in the world outside the host; or they may, like the trichina worm, be unable to live in this outer world. But whatever they do in these respects, they all have to use, not only a final host inside which their adult phases live and undergo sexual processes, but also an intermediate host, inside which the younger phases of their life histories must be parasitic. The parasitic younger phases, moreover, of most of the species here considered multiply their numbers inside the intermediate host and this is an important method by which parasitic animals increase their chances of survival in the world.

The Large Intestinal Fluke (Fasciolopsis buski)

This species is a flatworm that belongs to the Class of the phylum Platyhelminthes called the Trematoda or Flukes. The general shape and appearance of the adult fluke are shown in fig. 12. Its final hosts, in the small intestines of which the adults live, are man and the pig, though rarely they may be found in dogs. Rabbits can be infected experimentally, but all attempts to infect other animals have failed, so that this is a species with few final hosts. In man this fluke is found in China, Malaya, Borneo, and adjacent areas and also in Assam and Bengal. Stoll (1947) estimated that about 10 million people in the world were infected with this fluke at the time when he made his investigations.

74

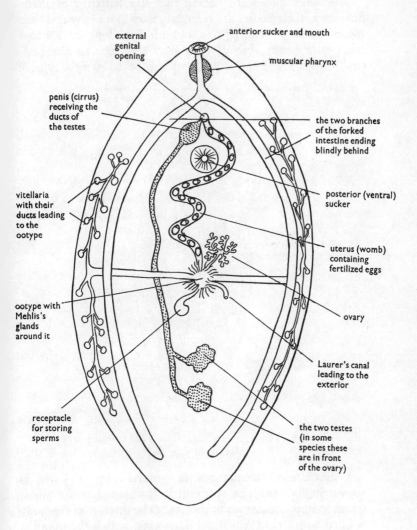

external genital opening

anterior sucker and mouth

muscular pharynx

penis (cirrus) receiving the ducts of the testes

the two branches of the forked intestine ending blindly behind

vitellaria with their ducts leading to the ootype

posterior (ventral) sucker

uterus (womb) containing fertilized eggs

ootype with Mehlis's glands around it

ovary

Laurer's canal leading to the exterior

receptacle for storing sperms

the two testes (in some species these are in front of the ovary)

Fig. 11. Diagram of the anatomy of a trematode worm (Fluke)

The adult flukes are not so thin and flattened as many flukes are; their bodies are relatively thick and fleshy and they measure 2 to 7·5 cm. ($\frac{3}{4}$ to about 3 inches) long by 0·8 to 2 cm. ($\frac{3}{10}$ to $\frac{4}{5}$ inch) broad. They have therefore an elongate-oval shape. The internal anatomy can be taken as a type of

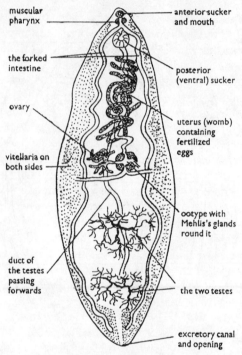

muscular pharynx

anterior sucker and mouth

the forked intestine

posterior (ventral) sucker

ovary

uterus (womb) containing fertilized eggs

vitellaria on both sides

ootype with Mehlis's glands round it

duct of the testes passing forwards

the two testes

excretory canal and opening

Fig. 12. The large intestinal fluke (*Fasciolopsis buski*). Hermaphrodite adult

the structure of trematodes in general (fig. 11). It is shown in fig. 12. The soft cuticle is covered with spines, which irritate the tissues of the host. The interior of the body is filled entirely, as it is in all flatworms, with a tissue called the *parenchyma*, in which all the organs are embedded. At the anterior end there is a mouth, surrounded by an anterior or *oral sucker*, closely behind which there is, on the ventral side, another, larger sucker, called the *ventral sucker*. In many flukes this ventral sucker is further back, nearer the middle of the body, or it may be at its posterior end. With the suckers the fluke holds on to the tissues of its host.

Some flukes have, in addition to suckers, hooks or clamps, with which they also hold on to the host, but these are absent from *Fasciolopsis buski*.

The mouth leads into a short pharynx or gullet and this leads into the intestine. The intestine of all flukes divides into two branches which run down the sides of the body. Both the branches end blindly near the posterior end of the body. There is, that is to say, no vent (anus), and this is another characteristic of flukes. There is a ring of nerve ganglia round the gullet, from which nerves pass into the body. The kidneys are represented by tubes in the body which have inside them cells provided with long protoplasmic processes (cilia) which project into the cavities of the tubes. These cilia create currents in the tubes and thus waft the waste material out of the body. Their movement looks rather like the flickering of a flame and these excretory cells are called *flame cells*. They are characteristic of the flatworms (tapeworms and flukes). All flukes, except those that belong to the family Schistosomatidae described below, are hermaphrodite, and the male and female sexual organs are voluminous and fill most of the body. The male sexual organs of *F. buski* consist of two branched *testes*, which produce sperms, and tubes which conduct these sperms to an organ called the *cirrus* which introduces them into the female genital opening; the female sexual organs include a more or less spherical *ovary*, which produces the eggs, a *shell-gland* and paired and numerous yolk glands (*vitellaria*), which together make the shells of the eggs and their yolk, and a branched tube, the womb or *uterus*, in which the fertilized eggs are stored. *Fasciolopsis buski* is, like many flukes, a prolific producer of eggs. It may produce 15,000 to 48,000 eggs a day.

The fertilized egg is 130 to 140 micra by 85 micra broad. It is yellowish-brown and has a thick, clear shell. At one end each egg has the lid (*operculum*), which is characteristic of the eggs of trematodes.

77

The life history of this species is shown in fig. 13. It resembles the life history of the liver fluke of sheep and cattle, *Fasciola hepatica*. The eggs are passed out in the excreta of the host and a small, ciliated *miracidium* develops in each of them. This is the first larval phase and all trematodes produce a first larva of this type. The miracidium swims in water with the cilia that cover its body. Its function is to find the intermediate host and enter its body to become parasitic inside it. Unless it does this within a few hours it will die. The intermediate host in this instance is an aquatic snail and usually the miracidium finds and enters the body of a snail within two hours of its liberation from the egg. Any snail will, of course, not do. It must be a snail belonging to the genera *Segmentina*, *Hippeutis* and *Gyraulus*, the commonest species used being *Segmentina hemisphaerula*, *Hippeutis cantori*, and *Hippeutis umbilicalis*. This species of fluke therefore has several possible intermediate hosts.

The miracidium either bores through the soft skin of the snail, or enters through the snail's respiratory opening, and, penetrating into its lymph spaces, becomes the next larval phase, which is called the *sporocyst*.

The sporocyst is a motile phase which contains germinal cells. It feeds on the tissues of the snail until it measures about 400×110 micra and then it moves to the heart and digestive gland of the snail. Inside it the next larval phase, which is called the *redia*, is produced by the germinal cells. The redia is a more elongate phase that has a food canal, germinal cells, and an opening through which its descendants are born. Numerous rediae are produced by each sporocyst, which ruptures to set them free. Each redia may then produce a number of daughter rediae. These daughter rediae then produce the next larval phase, which is practically a young fluke. It is called the *cercaria* and this is the phase which infects the final host. It corresponds, therefore, to the third infective larva of a hookworm or to the infective phase of any other species of parasitic animal.

The cercaria is, in general shape, somewhat like the young tadpole of a frog. It has a slender tail, about 500 micra ($\frac{1}{50}$

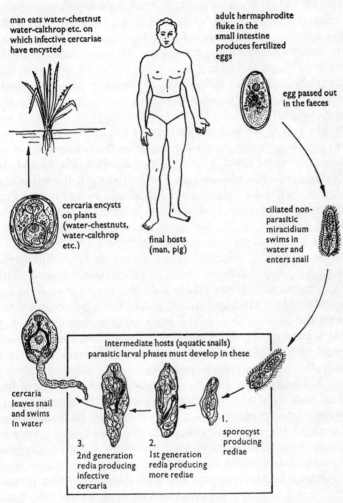

man eats water-chestnut water-calthrop etc. on which infective cercariae have encysted

adult hermaphrodite fluke in the small intestine produces fertilized eggs

egg passed out in the faeces

cercaria encysts on plants (water-chestnuts, water-calthrop etc.)

final hosts (man, pig)

ciliated non-parasitic miracidium swims in water and enters snail

Intermediate hosts (aquatic snails) parasitic larval phases must develop in these

cercaria leaves snail and swims in water

1. sporocyst producing rediae

3. 2nd generation redia producing infective cercaria

2. 1st generation redia producing more rediae

Fig. 13. Life history of the large intestinal fluke, *Fasciolopsis buski*

inch) long and a relatively heavy body which measures about 195 by 145 micra. The body, like the body of the adult fluke which the cercaria will become when it enters the final host, has a mouth leading into a forked food canal, a sucker round its mouth (oral sucker), and another on the ventral surface of its body (ventral sucker). It also has excretory organs in the form of flame cells and glands (*cystogenous glands*), which make the walls of the protective cyst in which it will presently enclose itself.

The cercaria leaves the snail and swims for a while in the water with its tail, or crawls along the leaves and stems of aquatic plants. Then it settles down on these plants and its cystogenous cells enclose it in a protective cyst, the tail being then cast off. Each cyst measures about 216 by 187 micra. The cercariae may encyst on almost any water plant, but the plants most likely to enable the cercariae to infect man are such edible water plants as the water calthrop (*Trapa natans, T. bispinosa,* and *T. bicornis*), the water hyacinth (*Eichhornia crassipes*), and the water chestnut (*Eliocharis tuberosa*). The fruit, bulbs, and stems of these and other plants are sold in the markets of the East and are eaten raw, often by peeling them with the teeth. The cercarial cysts are then ruptured by the teeth and the cercariae inside them are swallowed into the food canal of man. The cercariae can, of course, reach the plants only from infected snails and these can be infected only by miracidia derived from eggs passed out in the excreta of the final hosts, namely, man and the pig and the dog. The red water calthrop often carries many cercariae, because human faeces may be used to fertilize this plant when it is grown in ponds. Infection can be avoided, therefore, by not eating the aquatic plants unless they have been cooked or unless they have been dried, for drying kills the cercariae. A more certain method of avoiding infection, however, is to get rid of the snails that are the intermediate hosts. This unfortunately is not an easy task.

Stoll (1947) estimated that about 10 million people in the world were infected with this species at the time when he made his investigations. It causes inflammation of the wall of the small intestine to which the flukes attach themselves and ulceration of this part of the food canal; or bleeding from it may occur. When large numbers of the flukes are present – and over 3,000 of them have been recovered from a child of 9 – the effects may be severe. People may go on infecting themselves by eating water calthrops when they are working in the fields. They suffer chiefly from abdominal pain, diarrhoea, anaemia, and collections of fluid in the abdomen or under the skin (oedema and anasarca). The abdomen may therefore become distended and the patient may become very ill and may die.

Apart from the fact that this life history is indirect, the parasitic animal being compelled to develop, during its younger stages, inside an intermediate host, inside which it produces a phase, the cercaria, which infects the final host, we note, for comparison with other life histories, the following points:

1. There are virtually only two final hosts, namely the pig and man, the dog being only rarely infected with this parasite.
2. There are only a few species of snails that can act as intermediate hosts.
3. The infective phase of the parasite, the cercaria, is actually eaten by the final host. It is, moreover, a passive phase, enclosed in a cyst, and it must wait in this until it is eaten by the final host. It is, however, active before it assumes this passive phase and, while it is active, it places itself in a position in which it is likely to be eaten by the final host.
4. The parasite, during its development inside the intermediate host, multiplies the number of individuals derived from each of the fertilized eggs. Each egg, that is to say, gives origin to only one miracidium, and this, when it enters the snail, becomes a single sporocyst. But from each sporocyst numerous rediae arise, and by each of these more rediae may be formed. As if this were not enough, each redia produces numerous cercariae. The parasite's chances of infecting the final host are in this manner greatly increased.

Many other species of parasitic animals that have indirect

81

life histories multiply, inside their intermediate hosts, the numbers of infective phases derived from each fertilized egg. They may be contrasted with such species as the nematode hookworms, and, indeed, the roundworms generally, each fertilized egg of which gives origin, not to many, but to only one infective phase. The rate of infection with roundworms, is therefore likely to be slower than it is with species whose infective phases are multiplied inside an intermediate host. Multiplication of infective phases may not be an unqualified advantage for the parasitic animal; but it does increase the chances of the survival of the species in the struggle for life.

Another difference between the hookworm and the fluke is the fact that the fertilized egg of the hookworm can give rise, even under the most favourable circumstances, only to a single adult worm; and this worm must be either a female or a male. The success of two infective phases at least is therefore required if both a male and female are to survive to continue the species by sexual reproduction in the host. Each fertilized egg of the fluke, on the other hand, gives origin to many adult worms; and each of these is hermaphrodite, so that male and female survive in each individual.

There are other flukes parasitic in man which have life histories similar to that of the large intestinal fluke. Man is a normal host of some of these, but by others he is more rarely or only occasionally infected. It is not possible to describe all these species in this book, but the following three species are examples of them:

Fasciola hepatica

This species (Plate 1a) is the common liver fluke of cattle, sheep, rabbits, and other mammals. Its life history has been outlined in chapter 2 and is illustrated in fig. 4. The cercaria, derived from aquatic or amphibious snails which are the intermediate hosts, swims in water and eventually encysts on grass or water plants and is eaten by sheep, cattle, or the other final hosts. Man may eat them when they get on to salad plants, such as watercress, which are eaten uncooked, or when they get on to fruit that falls into water in which the cercariae are swimming. In the Lebanon and Armenia, where the people eat the raw livers of sheep and goats infected with the adult flukes, the flukes may temporarily adhere to the lining of the throat, larynx, and nasal passages, causing swelling and difficulty of swallowing or breathing and similar symptoms. This affliction is called *halzoun*. It must be differentiated from infection of the throat with the leech, *Limnatis nilotica*, described in chapter 10. In sheep and cattle and hosts other than man, the young flukes, when they reach the liver, burrow in this organ and cause extensive damage and eventually settle in the bile ducts, where they cause thickening of these ducts. Acute infections with them may kill sheep quickly; but usually the disease (*fascioliasis*) is more chronic. In man the flukes may also damage the liver and bile ducts and poisonous substances produced by them add to the injury caused. Among the symptoms produced are liver colic, abdominal pain, vomiting, and anaemia. When only a few flukes are present, the illness may be mild and it is then diagnosed only with difficulty.

Gastrodiscoides hominis

This species is fairly common in man in Assam and Cochin China. Stoll (1947) calculated that only a few hundred people in the world were infected with it at the time when he made his investigations. It is a small, reddish, pear-shaped fluke, about 5 mm. long and about 8 mm. broad. Its anterior end is conical and its posterior end is expanded and shaped somewhat like a saucer. Its life history is not known, but its relatives use snails as their intermediate hosts. It belongs to a family of flukes (Paramphistomidae) the members of which have the ventral sucker at the posterior end of the body. It also infects the pig, which is a common reservoir host.

Echinostoma ilocanum

This species may be found in man in the Philippine Islands and the islands in the South Pacific Ocean. It belongs to a family of flukes (Echinostomatidae) the members of which have, round the mouth, a disc provided with spines. Species of this family also use snails as their intermediate hosts. Human beings infect themselves by eating raw snails that are infected with the cercariae. The adult flukes attach themselves to the lining of the small intestine and cause intestinal colic and diarrhoea. There are other species of this genus that may infect man in the South Pacific area, but the exact identities of these species are still under discussion.

We have now seen, in chapters 3 and 4, that there are, among parasitic animals with direct life histories, species, such as the large roundworm, *Ascaris lumbricoides*, which can infect a host only through its mouth; and others, such as the hookworms, which, although they can infect a host through its mouth, normally enter it through its skin. Among parasitic animals with indirect life histories we find parallels to these two routes of infection. The large intestinal fluke just described and the tapeworms and flukes described in chapters 6 and 7, are examples of species with indirect life histories which infect their hosts through the mouth; and the rest of this chapter will describe two kinds of parasitic animals with indirect life histories which infect their hosts through the skin. These are the flukes belonging to the genus *Schistosoma*, which live in the blood of man and the roundworms that cause the disease called filariasis.

THE BLOOD-FLUKES OF MAN

The species of flukes (Trematoda) that are called blood-flukes are flukes which live, not in the food canal, liver, or other organs, but in the blood vessels of their hosts. They all belong to the family Schistosomatidae and the species of this family differ from all other flukes in one important respect – they are all unisexual, so that both males and females are found. This fact, together with the fact that these species normally enter their final hosts through the skin, although they can also enter these hosts through the mouth, differentiates the blood-flukes from other trematodes.

Three species of blood-flukes may infect man, in whom they cause the disease called *schistosomiasis*. Man is infected with these three species for the most part in the tropical areas of the world. One of the three, *Schistosoma haematobium*, affects chiefly the urinary bladder of man, and man is practically its only final host; another, *Schistosoma mansoni*, affects chiefly the large intestine, and man is also practically the only final host of this species; the third species, *Schistosoma japonicum*, affects chiefly the small intestine of man and it is confined to certain areas in Japan, China, and adjacent areas in the Far East; its final hosts include not only man, but also other mammals, among which are animals cultivated or kept as pets by man, such as cattle, water-buffalo, sheep, goats, dogs, and cats, so that man, who is constantly in contact with these other hosts, may acquire infection with this blood-fluke from them. The intermediate hosts of all these three species are aquatic snails.

The Urinary Blood-Fluke (*Schistosoma haematobium*)

The life history of this species is shown in fig. 14. The principal natural final host is man, although the mangabey monkey (*Cercocebus torquatus atys*) has been found naturally infected. Human infections therefore come practically always from other human beings. Stoll (1947) estimated that, at that time, about 39 million people in the world were infected with this species. Berberian *et al.* (1953) concluded from observations on a male patient that *S. haematobium* and *S. mansoni* can live in man for 26, and perhaps for 40, years.

The geographical distribution of *S. haematobium* is naturally the same as that of the intermediate hosts on which it depends for completion of its life history. This is, of course, true of all species with indirect life histories. *Schistosoma haematobium* infects man in Africa, Southern Europe, Palestine, Syria, Arabia, and Iraq. In Southern Europe it occurs in more or less isolated areas in Spain, Portugal, Greece, and Cyprus. In Africa it extends along the Mediterranean from Morocco to Egypt, down through Egypt and the Sudan to East and Central Africa as far as Rhodesia and South Africa; it also occurs in the Belgian Congo and in West Africa from the coast inland to Lake Tchad and the Upper Niger areas and also in Angola; it is also found in Madagascar and Mauritius. Pos-

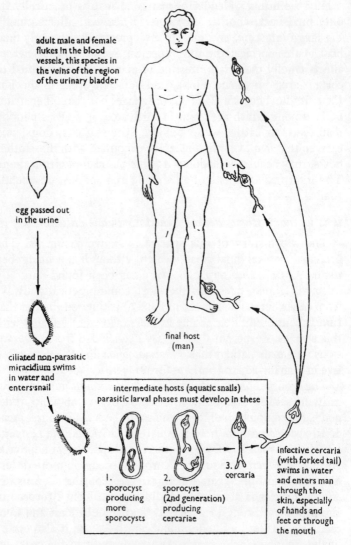

adult male and female flukes in the blood vessels, this species in the veins of the region of the urinary bladder

egg passed out in the urine

ciliated non-parasitic miracidium swims in water and enters snail

final host (man)

intermediate hosts (aquatic snails) parasitic larval phases must develop in these

1. sporocyst producing more sporocysts

2. sporocyst (2nd generation) producing cercariae

3. cercaria

infective cercaria (with forked tail) swims in water and enters man through the skin, especially of hands and feet or through the mouth

Fig. 14. Life history of the urinary blood-fluke, *Schistosoma haematobium*

sibly this species began to infect man in the Nile Valley and spread from this area to other parts of Africa. In man it has been parasitic for a very long time. Evidences of the disease it causes have been found in Egyptian mummies.

The elongated adult flukes (fig. 15) live chiefly in the veins of the urinary bladder of man, although some of them may live

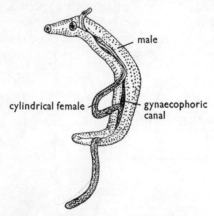

Fig. 15. Adults blood-flukes of the genus *Schistosoma*, showing the male holding the cylindrical female in the gynaecophoric canal

in the veins which collect blood from the food canal and take it to the liver (hepatic portal veins) or even in other veins. The male fluke is 10 to 15 mm. ($\frac{2}{5}$ to $\frac{1}{2}$ inch) long and 0·8 to 1 mm. ($\frac{8}{100}$ to $\frac{1}{25}$ inch) broad. The female is about 20 mm. ($\frac{3}{4}$ inch) long and 0·25 mm. ($\frac{1}{100}$ inch) in diameter.

When the male is fertilizing the female, its body is folded to form a groove, called the *gynaecocophoric canal*, inside which the cylindrical body of the female is held (fig. 15). This is a good example of the interesting adaptations made by parasitic animals to facilitate or ensure the success of sexual reproduction. When fertilization is not in progress the males and females may be found separated from one another.

The fertilized eggs are laid by the female into the small veins of the urinary bladder or, less often, into other small veins near by. When the small vein is filled with eggs the female worm moves to another small vein and fills that. The total number of eggs laid by the female during her life is not known with certainty, but it must be considerable, because this species of the genus *Schistosoma* may live in man for 26 to 40 years (see above). It is unlikely, however, that the female worm produces eggs throughout this period, or that she produces them at the same rate throughout her egg-laying period.

The injury done to the host is inflicted chiefly by the fertilized eggs. The eggs must leave the host and their nearest way

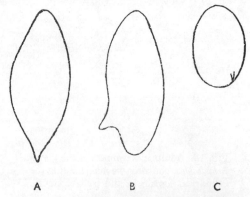

A   B   C

Fig. 16. Eggs of the three species of blood-flukes (*Schistosoma*) parasitic in man. A, egg of *Schistosoma haematobium*; B, egg of *Schistosoma mansoni*; C, egg of *Schistosoma japonicum*

out to the exterior is through the wall of the bladder into the urine, which is voided by the host. This is, in fact, the route they take and it is a route only rarely used by any kind of parasitic animal. No other animal parasitic in man uses this route out of the host. It involves an actual break through the walls of the bladder and this somewhat difficult operation is aided by two features of the egg.

Each egg (fig. 16A) has a light yellowish-brown transparent shell and at one end of it there is a pointed spine. The whole egg measures 112 to 170 micra long by 40 to 70 micra broad. In it, when the egg is laid, there is a miracidium, so that this species protects the development of its youngest larval stage inside the body of the host. The two features of the egg, however, that help it to get out of the host through the walls of the urinary bladder are: (1) its terminal spine; this irritates the tissues of the host so that muscular contractions of these occur which slowly expel the egg through the tissues of the bladder wall; (2) digestive juices, produced by the egg; these ooze out of the egg and dissolve the tissues around it, so that its passage through them is made easier. A combination of these two factors, the muscular contraction of organs into which the eggs pass, and the digestive action of substances produced by the egg, together with other factors which cannot be fully described here, enable the egg to pass slowly through the tissues of the host surrounding the small veins into which the eggs are laid. Because the eggs are laid chiefly in the small veins of the urinary bladder, they pass in this manner through the bladder walls and into the urine that the bladder holds. In this they are voided out of the host and thus reach the exterior.

The passage of the eggs through the bladder wall is not, however, effected without resistance to their passage by the host. The host's tissues react to these spined and irritating eggs just as they do to other invaders of the host's body. The eggs are attacked by phagocytes; the tissues around them become inflamed and the host attempts to enclose and immobilize them in capsules of fibrous tissue. The walls of the bladder therefore become inflamed and eventually overgrown and thickened by chronic inflammation. Finger-like growths into the bladder (papillomata) may result, and pain and bleeding may occur when the spined eggs are passed out in the urine. A whole series of symptoms, all referable to disturbances of the bladder and its functions, may therefore be shown by the infected person at this time. Other symptoms may be caused by poisonous substances produced by the worms themselves and may precede the symptoms caused by the passage of the eggs to the exterior.

The eggs hatch when they reach the exterior of the host and the miracidium in each of them is set free. Like other miracidia, it can live for only a few hours and it dies if it does not encounter one of the intermediate hosts. The intermediate hosts of *Schistosoma haematobium* are aquatic snails, not provided with opercula to close up the shell, which belong chiefly to the genera *Bulinus* and *Physopsis*. The species of these genera that are used by *S. haematobium* differ in different parts of the world and it is claimed that, in some areas, species of the genus *Planorbis* and perhaps also species of one or two other genera can also act as intermediate hosts.

When it meets a suitable snail the miracidium bores its way into it and becomes, just as the miracidium of the large intestinal fluke does, the *sporocyst* stage (fig. 17A). The sporocyst does not, however, produce rediae. None of the species of the family Schistosomatidae produce rediae, and in this respect they differ from the other flukes described in this book. The redia stage is missed out. The sporocyst produces, instead of rediae, a second generation of sporocysts and these directly produce cercariae.

The cercariae also provide a feature which is characteristic of all the species of the family of Schistosomatidae. Their tails are forked in the manner shown in fig. 17B. The cercaria of *Schistosoma haematobium* (fig. 17B) has an elongated, ovoid body which measures 140 to 240 by 57 to 100 micra. The single trunk of its forked tail is 175 to 250 micra long and each of the forks on this is 60 to 100 micra long. The whole tail is thus nearly twice as long as the body. The cercariae swim very strongly up and down in the water, the tail going first, and sometimes they attach themselves to various objects by means of their ventral suckers. If a human being washes his hands, or bathes any part of his skin in water containing the cercariae, any cercaria coming in contact with the skin may penetrate the skin. They may also penetrate the lining of the mouth if water containing them is used for drinking or washing the mouth. They penetrate the skin by forcing the anterior end against the skin and softening the skin by means of digestive fluids secreted by glands inside the cercaria. As it enters the skin the cercaria casts off its tail and it then makes its way to the small veins in the skin. It can reach these in 20 to 24 hours after it began to enter the skin. The entry into the skin may cause irritation and small haemorrhages somewhat resembling the lesions caused by flea bites, but these usually disappear in a day or two.

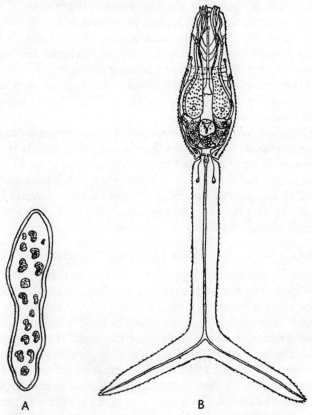

Fig. 17. Larval forms of a human blood-fluke (*Schistosoma*). (A) sporocyst; (B) cercaria with its forked tail

When they have reached the small veins in the skin, the cercariae are carried by the venous blood to the right side of the heart, from which they pass on to the lungs, in the capillaries of which they may be held up for a few days; but soon they pass on with the oxygenated blood to the left side of the heart and thus they reach the general arterial circulation. In this they pass all over the body, but the only ones that survive are the ones that enter the mesenteric artery that takes arterial blood to the liver. In the liver the cercariae, which are now young flukes, grow and become sexually mature. Then they move from the liver, against the stream of blood coming to the liver from the abdominal organs, to the veins in the pelvis and especially those of the bladder, in which the adult flukes are usually found. They usually arrive in the veins of the bladder region from one to three months after the cercaria penetrated the skin, but they may become sexually mature some time earlier.

The effects of *Schistosoma haematobium* have been indicated during the description of the life history just given. It is not necessary to refer to them further in this book, except to remind the reader that the chief injury done to the final host is done, as the injury done by the Guinea worm, described in chapter 6, also is, when the parasite, in the form of its spined eggs, is leaving the host.

The Intestinal Blood-Fluke (*Schistosoma mansoni*)

The life history of this species is similar to that of *Schistosoma haematobium*, except that the adult flukes settle down, not in the veins of the urinary bladder, but in those of the large intestine. The eggs, (fig. 16B), which have a lateral spine, therefore pass out of the host through the walls of the intestine and leave the host in its faeces. As they pass out they cause damage, and reactions of the host, similar to those caused by *S. haematobium*, but the damage is done, not to the bladder, but to the intestinal wall. The symptoms of the disease are therefore referable to the food canal rather than to the urinary system.

The intestinal blood-fluke, like the urinary blood-fluke, uses man only as its principal final host; but monkeys have been found naturally infected. Stoll (1947) estimated that, at the time when he made his investigations, about 29 million people in the world were infected with this species of fluke. It infects man in Africa and northern South America, but it does not occur in Europe. In Africa its distribution overlaps that of *S.*

haematobium to some extent. It is found in Egypt and down through eastern and central Africa to Northern Rhodesia and South Africa; in the Belgian Congo and in West Africa in Senegal and inland to French equatorial Africa and Lake Tchad; and also in Madagascar. It has been found in the south-western tip of Arabia. In South America it occurs in Brazil, Venezuela, Dutch Guiana, and the West Indies. Probably it was brought to South America by African slaves and succeeded in finding suitable snail intermediate hosts in its new South American habitat. It will be remembered that the hookworm, *Necator americanus,* probably reached North America in the same manner, but it had there an easier task in maintaining itself, because it does not require an intermediate as well as a final human host.

The adult male of *S. mansoni* is 6·4 to 9·9 mm. long and the adult female 7·2 to 14 mm. long. The two sexes are found in the small veins that collect blood from the large intestine and lowermost portion of the small intestine, and here they lay their eggs. They may live in man for at least twenty-six years. Each egg is about the same size as the egg of *S. haematobium*, and, like the egg of that species, it contains a miracidium when it is laid, but the spine on it comes out of the side of the egg near one end. These eggs with lateral spines make their way, much as those of *S. haematobium* do, out of the small veins, but they then find themselves, not in the wall of the bladder, but in the wall of the large intestine and rectum. Through this they make their way, causing, as they go, inflammation and reactions of the host's tissues similar to those caused by the eggs of *S. haematobium* in the wall of the bladder. The result is that the intestinal wall becomes thickened and fibrosed and its functions are disturbed. Ulcers inside the bowel may be found when the eggs break through into the contents of this part of the food canal. In addition, some of the eggs may be carried by the blood to the liver and may cause inflammation and fibrosis there. They may also be carried by the blood to other organs, such as the spleen, the lungs, the kidneys, the heart and spinal cord, where they also cause chronic inflammation. The main symptoms of infection with this species are, therefore, intestinal and hepatic. The infected person suffers from abdominal pain and dysentery, and finger-like growths (papillomata) of the lining of the large intestine may be formed. The liver and spleen are often greatly enlarged and inflamed and may be full of eggs.

The rest of the life history of this species resembles that of *Schistosoma haematobium*. The miracidia escape from the eggs outside the host and penetrate into the intermediate hosts, which are aquatic snails. The snails involved are, however, different. In Africa they belong to the genera *Planorbis, Biomphalaria, Physopsis,* and *Bulinus*; in the West Indies and South America they belong to the genera *Australorbis* and *Tropicorbis*.

Inside these snails the miracidia become sporocysts, each of which produces 200 to 400 daughter sporocysts. The daughter sporocysts then directly produce cercariae, which leave the snail and penetrate the skin of man, much as those of *Schistosoma haematobium* do. The daughter sporocysts may go on producing cercariae for several days or weeks and the number of cercariae produced by this species may be remarkable. It has been estimated that a single miracidium may, by producing sporocysts and daughter sporocysts, which then produce cercariae, produce as many as 3,500 cercariae a day for a considerable time, and that the total number of cercariae thus derived, during a period of months, from a single miracidium, may be 100,000 to 250,000. The chances of infecting man are thus enormously increased; and because each of these cercariae could, if it penetrated the skin of man, become a male or female adult fluke, the possible degree of human infection is correspondingly increased.

The Oriental Blood-Fluke (*Schistosoma japonicum*)

An important difference between this species and the other two species of human blood-flukes is the fact that man is by no means its only final host. Natural infections with it occur also in cattle, water-buffalo, horses, sheep, goats, dogs, cats, pigs, rats, and mice. Human infections with it are therefore not always derived from man, but may come from snails infected by eggs derived from any of these animals. Stoll (1947) estimated that about 46 million people in the world were infected with this species at the time when he made his investigations.

A second important difference between this species and the other two is that its geographical distribution is, as its name implies, limited to certain areas only in the Far East. It is found only in China, Japan, Formosa, Celebes, and the Philippine Islands.

The life history of this species resembles that of the two species of the genus *Schistosoma* just described, but the snails involved are again different. They are operculate snails belonging to the genus *Oncomelania*, which occur only in the Far East. Another difference in the life history is that the adult worms of this species live in the veinules of the small intestine, not in those of the large intestine or bladder. The eggs (fig. 16c), are oval and have, nearer one pole, a very small, blunt spine, which is usually seen only when the egg is in a certain position. These eggs are laid into the small veins in the wall of the small intestine and they accumulate there. Eventually they escape into the cavity of the small intestine, causing, as they do so, injury and inflammation of the intestinal wall. They then pass out with the excreta. Many eggs are, however, carried in the blood to the liver, spleen, and other organs, in which they cause inflammation and fibrosis. The infected person usually suffers from the disease in three stages. The first stage, called Katayama disease, lasts for about a month after infection and during it the parasites are invading the host and laying eggs; the infected person then suffers from a skin rash, abdominal pain, cough and other symptoms. In the second stage the patient suffers from dysentery, emaciation, and marked enlargement of the liver and spleen; these symptoms increase during the third stage, which occurs some 3 to 5 years after infection, and are accompanied by graver symptoms which usually end in death.

It is not necessary at this stage to discuss further the life histories of the three species of blood-flukes that infect man. It will be clear that they follow the general plan of the life history of the human intestinal fluke, except that the cercaria is able to infect the final host by penetrating its skin.

Animals Parasitic in Man

The development of the fluke inside its intermediate host also differs, the redia stage being omitted. Instead the sporocyst produces a second generation of sporocysts. The remarkable number of cercariae that may be produced inside the snail intermediate host has been indicated in the account of the life history of *Schistosoma mansoni*.

Bancroft's Filarial Worm (*Wuchereria bancrofti*)

This species is a roundworm belonging to the Order of roundworms called the Filarioidea, a name which refers to the fact that typical species of the Order are long, threadlike worms. They all have indirect life histories. The life history of Bancroft's filarial worm is shown in fig. 18.

The adult worm of this species lives in the lymphatic glands and in the lymphatic vessels that conduct the lymph from the tissues of the body, through the lymphatic glands, to the blood. Bancroft's filarial worm has only one final host, namely man, and it causes in him the disease called filariasis, one of the later manifestations of which may be the distressing and crippling enlargement of some parts of the body called elephantiasis. This disease, and the worms that cause it, are found in man in most of the tropical and subtropical parts of the world. It is difficult to differentiate infections with this species from infections with its relative *Brugia malayi* mentioned below, and often the same person is infected with both these species; but Stoll (1947) estimated that these two species infected, at the time when he made his investigations, about 189 millions of people in the world. In Europe *W. bancrofti* occurs around Barcelona in Spain, in Southern France, and in parts of the Balkans; in Africa along the Mediterranean and the East and West Coasts, but less often in the interior of Africa; in Asia it occurs along the coasts of Arabia, and in India, Malaya, China, Southern Korea, and Japan. It also occurs in the Dutch East Indies and South Pacific Islands, extending down to the northern coast of Australia. In South America it occurs in the West Indies and along the coast of South America from Northern Brazil to Colombia. Its distri-

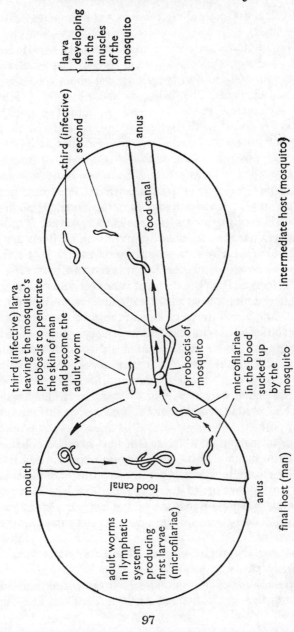

larva developing in the muscles of the mosquito

third (infective)
second

food canal

anus

third (infective) larva leaving the mosquito's proboscis to penetrate the skin of man and become the adult worm

proboscis of mosquito

microfilariae in the blood sucked up by the mosquito

intermediate host (mosquito)

mouth

food canal

anus

final host (man)

adult worms in lymphatic system producing first larvae (microfilariae)

Fig. 18. Life history of Bancroft's filarial worm, *Wuchereria bancrofti*

bution is thus chiefly along the coasts of the countries in which it is found.

The adult worms are creamy, threadlike nematodes that look like lengths of coarse sewing thread. The females are 65 to 100 mm. ($2\frac{1}{2}$ to 4 inches) long and about 0·25 mm. ($\frac{1}{100}$ inch) in diameter. The males are about 40 mm. ($1\frac{1}{2}$ inches) long and their diameter is about 0·1 mm. ($\frac{1}{250}$ inch). The adults are found in the lymphatic glands and vessels and in these situations the female lays, not eggs, but living first larvae, 225–300 micra long with a diameter of 10 micra. Each larva is called a *microfilaria* and the microfilarial larvae of this species are enclosed in delicate sheaths. They pass from the lymph into the blood and appear in the blood circulating near the surface of the body – in, that is to say, what is called the peripheral circulation, only during the night. They are found in the blood chiefly between the hours 10 p.m. to 4 a.m. This *nocturnal periodicity* of these larvae is shown also by relatives of this species and the reason for it is not certainly known. Various theories have been advanced to account for it, but none of them explains all the facts. One of the difficulties is that, when a person infected with these larvae sleeps by day and is active by night, or travels halfway round the world, the microfilarial larvae change the time when they appear in the peripheral blood; they then appear by day and not at night. It seems, therefore, that they appear in the peripheral blood when the infected person is inactive or asleep, whether this is so by day or by night.

The microfilariae, which are the first larvae, cannot develop further in the final host. They are removed from human blood by the mosquitoes which are the intermediate hosts and in these they develop to the third infective larval stage. It is tempting to suppose that the microfilariae appear in the peripheral blood of man at night because they then have better chances of being sucked up by the mosquitoes, which suck human blood at night; but this theory does not account for all the known facts.

The species of mosquitoes which can act as intermediate hosts of this species belong to the genera *Culex*, *Aedes*, and

Anopheles. About forty-one species of these genera can act in this way, so that this species, although it has only one final host, has a wide selection of intermediate hosts.

Inside the mosquitoes the development of the larvae resembles that undergone by the larvae of the hookworms described in chapter 3. The larval development of this filarial worm occurs, however, under the protection of the mosquito's body, while that of the hookworm larvae occurs outside the host.

What actually happens is that the first microfilarial larva passes to the muscles of the mosquito and there becomes the second larva, which develops, in the same situation, into the third infective larva. This development takes from 10 days to 2 weeks, and many microfilariae fail to become infective larvae. The infective larva then leaves the muscles of the mosquito and passes to its proboscis. When the mosquito sucks human blood, the infective larva breaks through the thin membrane covering part of the lower lip of the mosquito and thus gets on to the skin of man. It then either enters the wound made by the mosquito or gets in through some other wound in the skin. Experts seem to be agreed that the microfilariae cannot actively penetrate the unbroken skin. If, moreover, the weather is such that the skin of man is dry, the infective larvae are quickly killed by drying. Infection is therefore most likely to occur in hot weather, when the skin is moist. When they have entered the skin, the infective larvae find their way, by some route that is unknown, to the lymphatic vessels, in which they become adult male and female worms. The time required for this later development is not known with accuracy, but it is probably a period of several months. One reason why some time is required before a new generation of first microfilarial larvae can be produced, is the fact that males and females must mature and meet and fertilization of the females must occur. The adult worms live in man for about four or five years.

The disease caused by Bancroft's filarial worm is one variety of the disease called *filariasis*, which is caused by worms of this type. All the filarial worms tend to cause a slowly-developing chronic inflammation of the organs in which they live and this usually goes on for a period of years. Bancroft's filarial worm, because it lives in the lymphatic system of man, causes inflammation of this system.

About 10 to 22 months after being infected with the worms, or, in some instances, as early as 3 months after infection, the infected person experiences spells of pain in the part of the body in which the worms have settled down and there may be headache, backache, loss of appetite, and other symptoms of the inflammation of the lymphatic system. Lymphatic glands become swollen and often the genital organs are affected. Later on the course of the disease becomes chronic. The lymphatic glands become enlarged and the well-known enlargement of certain parts of the body called elephantiasis may develop. This is due to blocking of the lymphatic vessels and overgrowth of the connective tissues in the part of the body affected, which become swollen, sometimes to a monstrous size. Later the swollen parts become hard and liable to infection with bacteria. The genital organs and legs are often affected, so that gross deformities may result. Elephantiasis is, however, commoner among people who are over 30 years of age and in people who have lived for 30 years or more in areas in which the disease is common. Even in countries in which the disease is firmly established only about 1 to 5 per cent of infected people develop elephantiasis.

Other Filarial Worms Parasitic in Man

In India and Indonesia species of filarial worms formerly thought to be species of *Wuchereria* are parasitic in man, monkeys, tigers, dogs, cats, wild cats, and the loris, and some other mammals. These species have now been classified in the genus *Brugia*. Their intermediate hosts are mosquitoes belonging to the subgenus *Mansonoides* and to the genera *Anopheles* and *Aedes*. Their life histories resemble that of *Wuchereria bancrofti*, but only one of these species, namely, *Brugia malayi*, infects man, in whom it may be present together with Bancroft's filarial worm. The disease it causes resembles that caused by Bancroft's filarial worm, but the swelling (elephantiasis) affects the legs more often, and the genital organs are less often involved. The mosquito intermediate hosts of *Brugia malayi* breed chiefly in swamps and marshy districts and their larvae are attached to water plants, so that removal of these plants will help to reduce the numbers of the mosquitoes and therefore to control the infection. For the same reason infection with *Brugia malayi* is commoner in country districts, while infection with Bancroft's filarial worm is commoner in towns.

A species of filarial worm that lives, not in the lymphatic system of man, but in his connective tissues, especially in those of the skin, is *Onchocerca volvulus*. Man is its only final host. It is parasitic in man in Central Africa from Sierra Leone across to the Sudan and south to the Belgian Congo and Nyasaland. It also attacks man in Guatemala, southern Mexico, and north-west Venezuela, where workers on coffee plantations are often attacked. Possibly this filarial worm was originally brought to America by slaves imported from Africa and found, in its new habitat, suitable intermediate hosts. Stoll (1947) estimated that, at the time when he made his investigations, *Onchocerca volvulus* was present in about 20 million people in the world. Formerly it was thought that another species of the genus *Onchocerca* was also parasitic in man in America and this species was called *Onchocerca coecutiens*. It is now known that this species is, in fact, *O. volvulus*.

The life history of *Onchocerca volvulus* resembles that of Bancroft's filarial worm, but its intermediate hosts are not mosquitoes, but the small, blood-sucking insects related to the mosquitoes and gnats that are called blackflies (Simuliidae). These flies breed only in quickly-running steams, in which their remarkable aquatic larvae live. The species that act as intermediate hosts are, in Africa, *Simulium neavei* and a species appropriately called *Simulium damnosum* and, in Guatemala, Mexico, and the neighbouring areas, *Simulium ochraceum*, although *S. metallicum*, *S. callidum*, and perhaps other species are also intermediate hosts in some areas. *O. volvulus* is, therefore, confined, as Bancroft's worm is, to one species of final host, but can use more than one species of blackfly as its intermediate hosts.

Animals Parasitic in Man

The infective larva, when it enters the skin of man, migrates through the skin, or the tissues under the skin, and causes, as it does so, irritation and chronic inflammation. The result of this inflammation is that the worms become enclosed in fibrous tissue formed by the host, and lumps of this tissue, enclosing the worms, appear, underneath the skin. The lumps, which are called *nodules*, are usually 0·5 to 2·5 cm. ($\frac{1}{5}$ to 1 inch) in diameter, but they may be twice as big (5 cm.). Usually they take a year or longer to reach a diameter of 1 cm. They occur in people of all ages, babies and children included. Normally the nodules are painless and do not cause much trouble. The nodules may occur almost anywhere on the body, but in Africa they are commonest on the trunk, thighs, and arms, especially above the hips and on the elbows, knees, and ribs, and in Guatemala and Mexico, chiefly on the head and shoulders. This is probably associated with the type of clothing used, parts of the body that are not protected being more often bitten by the intermediate hosts. In Belgian Uele in Africa, for example, Europeans clothe the parts of the body below the waist, so that only 48 per cent of them were found to have nodules on this part of the body, whereas nodules were found in 88 per cent of the Africans, whose legs were uncovered. This cannot, however, be the whole explanation, because the infective larvae migrate away from the site at which they enter the human skin. The suggestion, formerly believed, that the distribution of the nodules is determined by the site at which the intermediate hosts bites, is not, therefore, entirely true. It has been suggested that the nodules occur more often at places where either the bones, or the clothing worn, apply pressure to the skin, so that the migrations of the infective larvae in the skin are impeded or held up. This might account for the fact that the nodules are common about the crests of the iliac bones and, in Guatemala and in parts of the Belgian Congo, on the head around the ears, where the brim of the hat constricts the skin.

While the nodules caused by *Onchocerca volvulus* are conspicuous effects of this species on man, it may have other effects, some of which are serious. The worms produce microfilariae, which migrate in the skin and cause inflammation of the skin. The skin may become thickened and wrinkled and purplish in colour, or there may be intense itching, accompanied by thickening of the skin; or there may be a disease somewhat like eczema. The microfilariae may also get into the lymphatic system, although they do not usually appear, as the microfilariae of Bancroft's filarial worm do, in the blood at the surface of the body. In the lymphatic glands, however, they cause inflammation and enlargement of the lymphatic glands and blocking of the flow of lymph may result. The consequence may then be that the tissues of the part affected may become waterlogged, so to speak, with lymph and may swell up, and elephantiasis may follow.

The most serious effects of infection with *Onchocerca volvulus* occur, however, when microfilarial larvae reach the eye and are held up in this organ. The inflammation that they then cause may inflict extensive damage on the eye and blindness is a frequent consequence. Usually this kind of injury to the eye is associated with numerous nodules on the head and it begins some seven to ten years after the sufferer was infected.

Although *Onchocerca volvulus* uses man only as its final host, it has relatives that cause similar disease in other animals. Among these relatives are *Onchocerca cervicalis*, which lives in the tissue of the strong ligament (*ligamentum nuchae*) that runs from the skull to the shoulders of the horse and mule. This species occurs in horses in Australia and England and probably elsewhere. Its intermediate host is the blood-sucking midge, *Culicoides nubeculosus*. There are other species of the genus *Onchocerca* which infect the fetlocks of horses and the nuchal ligament of cattle; and *Onchocerca gibsoni*, which lives in the connective tissues of the ox and zebu in Australia, India, Malaya, and South Africa, causes the formation of nodules in the beef, which make the parts affected unfit for human consumption; its intermediate host in Malaya is *Culicoides pungens*.

Another filarial worm parasitic in man in Central and West Africa is the eye-worm, *Loa loa*. The name 'eye-worm' has been given to this species because it may live in the anterior chamber of the eye, in front of the lens, and the worm may appear at times actually under the conjunctiva of the eye, where it can be seen moving along. It also, however, lives in the subcutaneous connective tissue in other parts of the body and may then cause swelling of the tissues around it. These swellings appear for a time in different places as the worm moves about, at a rate of about an inch in two minutes, and they are therefore called *fugitive swellings*, or Calabar swellings. They may be as big as a pigeon's or hen's egg.

Man is the only final host of this species, the life history of which is like that of Bancroft's filarial worm, except that the intermediate hosts are tabanid flies belonging to the genus *Chrysops*, which are related to the horse-flies and clegs. In West Africa the species involved are *Chrysops silacea* and *C. dimidiata* and, in Central Africa, *C. longicornis*, *C. distinctipennis*, and possibly also *C. centurionis*. Stoll (1947) estimated that, at the time when he made his investigations, about 13 million people in the world were infected with *Loa loa*.

The development of the infective larvae in these flies takes 10 to 12 days, the earlier larvae developing in the abdomen of the fly and the later stages in the head of the fly. These flies suck the blood of man by day and it is interesting to find that the microfilariae of *Loa loa*, which are sucked up by the bloodsucking flies, appear in the peripheral blood of man by day, not by night, as the microfilariae of Bancroft's filarial worm do. Like the infective larvae of Bancroft's filarial worm, the infective larvae of *Loa loa* break out of the proboscis of the fly and penetrate the skin of man. When they have entered the human body, the infective larvae require 3 to 4 years to develop into adult worms and the adult worms may live in man for 4 to 17 years. The whole infection therefore may last, if it is left alone, for many years.

Usually this species has comparatively little effect on man. As it wanders about in the subcutaneous tissues it causes the fugitive (Calabar) swellings which appear at irregular intervals and disappear again in a few days. Most often they appear on the hands or forearms or in the orbit, but they may appear on the back or chest or in the armpit or groin and in other parts of the body. The swellings are due to inflammation caused by the worm and are usually painless, apart from the itching and irritation that accompany them. When the worms settle in the region of the eye they cause irritation and swelling of the eyelids and, when the worm is in the anterior chamber of the eye, pain, secretion of tears, and disturbances of vision may occur. The worm may be seen underneath the conjunctiva or may move across the eye or across the bridge of the nose. When it does this it may be removed surgically.

Yet another species of filarial worm that may infect man is *Dipetalonema* (*Acanthocheilonema*) *perstans*, which may be parasitic in man in Africa from Senegal to British East Africa and south to Angola and the Zambezi valley. In South America it is found in Venezuela, Trinidad, the Guianas, Brazil, and Argentina. In addition to man, the chimpanzee and gorilla may be final hosts of this species and the intermediate hosts are the blood-sucking midges *Culicoides austeni* and *Culicoides grahami*. The adult worms are usually found alone and they do not cause much tissue reaction, so that they cause little trouble, although some experts think that they cause Calabar swellings and other effects. Stoll (1947) estimated that, at the time when he made his investigations, about 27 million people in the world were infected with *Dipetalonema perstans*.

In Panama, Colombia, northern Argentina, British and Dutch Guiana, and the islands St Vincent and Dominica, man may be the only final host of a filarial worm called *Mansonella ozzardi*, the intermediate host of which is the blood-sucking midge, *Culicoides furens*, and perhaps other midges belonging to this genus. These worms also have comparatively little effect on man. Stoll (1947) estimated that, at the time when he made his enquiries, about 7 million people in the world were infected with *Mansonella ozzardi*.

Related to the filarial worms described above are certain species that occur in dogs and other animals, but not in man. Among these is *Dirofilaria immitis*, the heartworm of the dog, which is also found in otters, cats, wild cats, and tigers. It lives in the heart of these hosts in Southern Europe, India, Japan, China, and North and South America. The intermediate hosts of this species are mosquitoes belonging to the genera *Anopheles*, *Aedes Myzorhynchus*, and *Culex*. These worms cause inflammation of the lining of the heart (endocarditis) or of the arteries, and clotting of the blood may result. If portions of the clots are detached and become lodged in the smaller arteries of the lungs, they may block up these arteries and a kind of pneumonia may then occur in the parts of the lung that are normally supplied with blood by the occluded arteries.

In horses all over the world, a species of the genus *Setaria*, *Setaria equina*, may be found in the abdominal cavity or the spaces round the lungs. Its intermediate host is the stable fly, *Stomoxys calcitrans*, which possibly also transmits *S. equina* to horses. A related species may occur in the abdominal cavity of cattle, antelope, and deer. Neither of these two species has serious effects on its hosts. A third species of this genus, *Setaria digitata*, is a parasite of the ox in Ceylon and Burma, to which it does little harm; but it may also be parasitic in sheep, goats, horses, and man and these unusual hosts may suffer more, as unusual hosts of other parasitic animals do. This species may get into the brain and spinal cord of horses and severe disease of the nervous system has been attributed to it; it has been accused of carrying the virus that causes a disease of the brain of horses and children in Japan. Another species, *Neurofilaria cornellensis*, has been found in the nervous system of sheep suffering from a disease of the nervous system.

Reviewing the life histories just described, we see that they follow the plan of the life histories of the blood-flukes described above, but there are two important differences. First, the infective larvae of the filarial worms do not have to wait, as the cercaria of the blood-flukes must, until they come into contact with the final hosts. They are carried to these hosts by the intermediate hosts; and their chances of reaching the final hosts are greatly increased by the fact that the intermediate hosts are urged to seek out the final hosts by one of the most powerful of the urges that govern the lives of all kinds of animals, namely, hunger. The intermediate host must have food and, as it gets it, it gives the filarial worm the opportunity to get into the body of its final host. The filarial worm, that is to say, uses, as its intermediate host, a species that is already a temporary parasite of the final host.

The second difference between the life histories of the filarial worms and the blood-flukes is the fact that the filarial worms have almost entirely got rid of the need to enter the world outside the host. They do not lay eggs; they produce living larvae, but this is also done by some species of parasitic animals that do enter the world outside the host. The mark of the life history of the filarial worms, and of other life histories that follow the same plan, is that the infective larvae produced by the female parasite are not equipped to withstand the effects of the world outside the host for longer than a few hours. They are quickly killed by drying and other factors outside the host. They are, in fact, protected inside the body of the intermediate host right up to the last minute, so to speak, right up to the moment when the intermediate host sucks the blood of the final host. Then, it is true, they must leave the intermediate host and brave the world outside it; but their stay in this injurious outer environment, which quickly kills them, need not last long. The intermediate host transports them to a position that is most favourable for their exit from the outer world into the body of the final host. We shall see, in the next three chapters, that some of the other animals parasitic in man which have indirect life histories have reduced to a minimum their stay in the world outside the host and that some of them, like the trichina worm among the species with direct life histories, have altogether eliminated the serious risk of entry into this world.

CHAPTER SIX

Animals Twice Parasitic in One Life
(CONTINUED)

THIS chapter and the next one will describe life histories during which the intermediate host is eaten by the final host, so that the infective larva has no need to leave the intermediate host and encounter the injurious influences of the world outside a host. Its eggs or first larvae have, however, still to enter the world outside a host. They must do this in order to get into the intermediate host. It is not until we consider, in chapter 8, the human malarial parasites, that we shall meet with a species that has eliminated altogether the need to enter the world outside a host.

As an example of a parasitic animal whose life history depends on the eating of the intermediate host, let us first consider the Guinea worm, *Dracunculus medinensis*.

The Guinea Worm (*Dracunculus medinensis*)

This nematode worm, which is perhaps the worm called, in the Bible, the 'fiery serpent', has infected man since the time of the Greek and Roman physicians and Galen gave the disease it causes the name *dracontiasis*. It is nowadays called, not only the Guinea worm, but also the Medina worm or the dragon worm. Stoll (1947) estimated that, in 1947, about 48 million people in the world were infected with the Guinea worm. It is found in Africa in the Nile Valley, in the central and equatorial regions of this continent and along its northwest and west coasts, and, in Asia, in Arabia, Persia, Afghanistan, Turkestan, and India. In central and western India as many as 25 per cent of the village people may be infected. The infection also occurs, but comparatively rarely, in the Dutch East Indies and south-eastern Soviet Russia. It has also been introduced into the West Indies, the Guianas, and the Bahia area of Brazil. Its life history is shown in fig. 19. Man is infected with it by swallowing its intermediate hosts, which are small Crustacea, all of which are species of the genus *Cyclops* (fig. 19).

The adult female worm, when she is mature, is a long, thin worm, measuring 500 to 1200 mm. (20 to 48 inches) long, but only 0·9 to 1·7 mm. ($\frac{1}{25}$ to $\frac{1}{14}$ inch) in diameter. The smaller male, which has only rarely been found, is only 12 to 29 mm. ($\frac{1}{2}$ to $1\frac{1}{2}$ inches) long. Both sexes live and mature in the connective tissues between the organs of the final hosts, which include man, dogs, wolves, foxes, cats, minks, and raccoons. They have also been found in monkeys, baboons, hares, cattle, and the leopard; but dogs seem to be less often infected than the other final hosts.

In dogs that have been experimentally infected the mature worms may be found in the connective tissues in the region of the shoulder blade or behind the gullet, or in the region of the groin, vertebral column, limbs, the wall of the chest and abdomen, the heart, or the eye. The male disappears soon after the female has been fertilized. The males have been found 15 to 20 weeks after the experimental infection of dogs, so that they live for at least as long as this. The female lives on in the connective tissues for about 10 to 14 months.

While the worms are living in the connective tissues of the host, the host seems not to be injured by the presence of the worms. At any rate, no symptoms of disease are caused. During all this time the female is maturing and producing, not fertilized eggs, but millions of active first larvae, which fill her womb (*uterus*). While these larvae are being produced the female ceases to feed and by the time that her womb has become filled with larvae, her food canal below the gullet has disappeared. Her body is now filled with the coils of her womb distended by the millions of larvae she has produced.

The female worm is now ready to discharge the larvae from her body. She does not, however, discharge them into the body of the final host, but into the world outside it: and to do

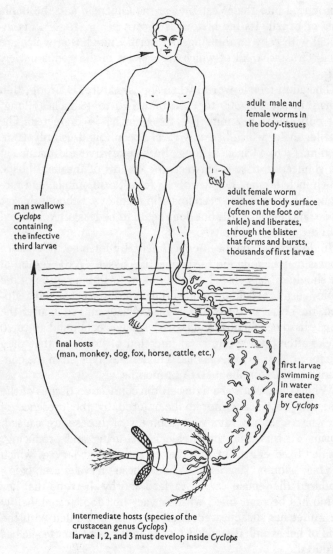

adult male and
female worms in
the body-tissues

adult female worm
reaches the body surface
(often on the foot or
ankle) and liberates,
through the blister
that forms and bursts,
thousands of first larvae

man swallows
Cyclops
containing
the infective
third larvae

final hosts
(man, monkey, dog, fox, horse, cattle, etc.)

first larvae
swimming
in water
are eaten
by *Cyclops*

intermediate hosts (species of the
crustacean genus *Cyclops*)
larvae 1, 2, and 3 must develop inside *Cyclops*

Fig. 19. Life history of the Guinea worm, *Dracunculus medinensis*

110

this she has to migrate to the surface of the final host. She may reach this at almost any point. In man, for instance, she may appear under the skin of the parts of the body that are likely to be immersed in cold water, such as the arms, breast, trunk or buttocks, or lower limbs; but she may cause blindness by developing in the orbit. Most often, however, she appears, in man, under the skin of the sole of the foot, or under the skin of the ankle. When she reaches the skin at any point the female worm may be seen or felt under the skin, where she may look like a small varicose vein. Her presence there causes a local reaction by the tissues of the host. This is shown by the appearance of localized reddening of the skin. There may also be, a few hours before this localized reaction occurs, itching, or a generalized rash with such symptoms as slight fever, nausea, vomiting, and diarrhoea, or asthma-like symptoms, or severe giddiness or syncope. It seems likely that these symptoms are due to liberation by the worm of substances that are poisonous to the host.

Ultimately the head of the worm comes near to the skin of the part of the body on which she points and, when this happens, or a few hours before it does, there is itching and a boring, burning, or dragging pain at this point. Then a small blister appears, which may reach a diameter of 2 to 6 cm. (up to $2\frac{1}{2}$ inches). If this blister is now immersed in cold water, it bursts and a small, shallow ulcer is seen beneath it, at the bottom of which there is a small hole. If this area is now douched with cold water, a milky fluid, containing thousands of the first larvae of the worm, is extruded from the hole in the skin, or a portion of the uterus of the worm is extruded through the hole and bursts in the water outside to liberate the larvae inside the womb of the worm.

In this manner the first larvae are set free into the water outside the host. Repeated douching of the area will 'milk' the uterus until all its larvae have been set free. The female worm of course dies during the process of liberating her brood.

The first larvae thus liberated from the womb of the worm are each about 500 to 750 micra ($\frac{1}{50}$ to $\frac{1}{33}$ inch) long. Each has a tail which constitutes about a third of the larva's length. They swim and coil about in the water and die there unless they are swallowed by the intermediate hosts, which are small freshwater Crustacea belonging to the genus *Cyclops* (fig. 19). Reaching the mid-gut of these Crustacea, the first larvae bore through the intestinal wall into the blood-space (haemocoel) around it, where they develop into infective larvae which are capable of infecting the final host again. This happens when man, or any of the other final hosts, swallow water containing *Cyclops* which contain the infective larvae. The digestive juices of the final host then digest the *Cyclops* and set free the infective larvae, which make their way from the food canal of the final host into the connective tissues of this host, where they grow up into the adult male and female worms.

In this life history there are, therefore, several different kinds of final hosts, but virtually only one genus of intermediate host, although numerous species of this genus can act as intermediate hosts.

Another feature of the life history is that the female worm produces, not eggs, but living first larvae. She is, that is to say, larviparous as the trichina worm, among the species with direct life histories, also is. Larviparity is, as we shall see, a feature of other parasitic animals; it is a feature of the tsetse flies, for example; and it helps, no doubt, to increase the chances of survival of the parasite, because the youngest phases of the life history are protected inside the body of the female parent, just as those of man and other mammals are. With it is no doubt correlated the remarkable method by which the female *Dracunculus* liberates her young from the host. We do not know how the female worm, at the end of a period of ten to fourteen months of life in the final host during which she causes no symptoms of disease, finds her way to the surface of the body of the host and usually to those points on its surface which are likely to be immersed in the water in which the intermediate host lives. But the feat performed by this female worm is certainly a remarkable one. No less remarkable is the fact that, when she has accomplished it, she provokes, for the first and only time in her life, tissue-reactions

112

Animals Twice Parasitic in One Life

in the final host, which liberate her young. The disease caused by this worm is therefore caused, as the disease caused by the blood-flukes considered in chapter 5 also is, when the parasite is liberating the young from the final host.

Another feature of the life history of the Guinea worm is that the parasite enters the world outside the host only once, namely, when it has left the final host and needs to enter the intermediate host. Once inside this it cannot do anything more to help itself. It cannot, as the cercaria of the liver-fluke can, move into a position in which it is likely to be swallowed by the final host. It must, like the tapeworms next to be described, wait until the final host swallows the body of the intermediate host in which it must remain.

TAPEWORMS

Tapeworms (Plate 1b) are, like the flukes described in chapter 5, flatworms belonging to the phylum Platyhelminthes, which includes the two classes *Cestoda* (Tapeworms) and *Trematoda* (Flukes). Flukes and tapeworms therefore have some characters in common, but there are also striking differences between them. Some of these differences are especially evident in species like the tapeworms described in this chapter and the fish-tapeworm described in chapter 7. One of the most obvious of these differences is the fact that, while the bodies of flukes consist of one piece only, the bodies of the majority of tapeworms are composed of a relatively small head, called the *scolex*, at the anterior end, and a chain of pieces, each of which is called a *segment* or *proglottis* (pl. *proglottides*). These segments arise from the scolex by a process of budding, which is called *strobilation* (*strobilization*). The chain of segments may be quite short, as it is, for example, in *Echinococcus granulosus* (fig. 27) described below, which has only 3 or 4 segments in the chain, or it may be up to 30 feet or more in length, as it is, for example, in the giant fish tapeworm of man, which has some 3,000 to 4,000 segments in the chain.

The head (*scolex*) is often small, or even minute, in comparison with the size of the segments and the length of the

113

whole chain of these. It has on its outer surface muscular suckers (Plate 2a) and sometimes *hooks* (fig. 20) as well and the tapeworm holds on to its host by means of these. There is no mouth on the head, because all tapeworms have lost, in the course of their adaptation to parasitic life, the entire food canal. They cannot therefore feed by taking food into their mouths. They absorb it, through the soft skin, from the contents of the food canal of the host, which provide them, so to speak, with a bath of food in which they are immersed. Inside the head are the principal nerve ganglia and from these longitudinal nerve cords run throughout the length of the

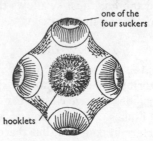

one of the
four suckers

hooklets

Fig. 20. Head of the pork tapeworm, *Taenia solium*

chain. All down the sides of the whole chain there are tubes, formerly called the *excretory canals*, which may have the function of removing waste materials; but some experts believe that they regulate the osmotic pressure of fluids in the tapeworm's body and for this reason they are nowadays often called *osmoregulatory canals*.

The existence of these organs which pass through the whole length of the tapeworm chain shows that the whole chain and its scolex constitute an individual. When, however, the segments are considered, it is clear that each segment is, so far as sexual reproduction is concerned, a separate individual.

The segments may be formed either directly from the scolex, or from a short and unsegmented portion of the worm called its *neck*, which immediately succeeds the scolex. After one segment has been formed, another is formed in front of it nearer the head, so that the segment first formed is pushed

114

further away from the head. By repetition of this process the length of the chain is increased. As the segments first formed move further and further away from the head they develop sexual organs. The male sexual organs (fig. 21) are formed before the female sexual organs appear. They consist of numerous *testes* scattered through the spongy tissue (*parenchyma*) of the solid segment, and a duct (*vas deferens*), which conducts the sperms made by the testes to an organ called the *cirrus*, which introduces them into the female genital opening. Frequently the cirrus and the male external genital opening is

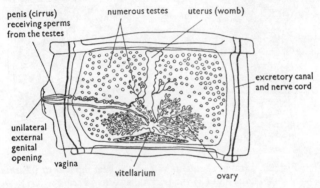

Fig. 21. A segment (proglottid) of the pork tapeworm,
Taenia solium

at the side of each segment. In the beef tapeworm (fig. 21) it opens on alternate sides of succeeding segments; in the fish tapeworm (fig. 33) it opens in the middle of each segment; in other tapeworms, such as the common tapeworm of the dog, *Dipylidium caninum* (fig. 26), there are two sets of male and female sexual organs in each segment and there are two male sexual openings, one on each side of each segment.

As the male sexual organs mature and produce sperms, the female sexual organs (fig. 21) begin to appear. These consist, as they do in flukes, of an external female genital opening, situated usually close to the male external genital opening, through which the sperms are introduced by the cirrus of the male; a *vagina*, which conducts the sperms to a sac (*receptaculum seminis*) in which the sperms are stored; an *ovary*, which produces eggs; and a sac called the *ootype*, into which the eggs pass to receive their yolk and shells made by the *shell-glands* and the yolk glands (*vitellaria*). The eggs then pass into the womb (*uterus*), the shape of which varies considerably in different tapeworms. In some species the eggs pass out of the womb into special sacs outside it called *egg-capsules* or *par-uterine* organs, in which the eggs are stored till they are liberated from the worm. The uterus of the beef tape-

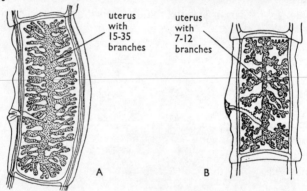

Fig. 22. Gravid segments of (A) the beef tapeworm (*Taenia saginata*) and (B) the pork tapeworm (*Taenia solium*)

worm (fig. 22A) is a straight tube, without an opening to the exterior, which runs up the middle of the segment and has 15 to 35 lateral branches on each side; the uterus of the pork tapeworm, *Taenia solium* (fig. 22B), is similar, but it has only 7 to 12 lateral branches on each side; the uterus of the fish tapeworm of man (fig. 33) is a rosette-shaped sac in the middle of each segment.

Because the male sexual organs develop before the female ones, the structure and appearance of the segments vary according to the degree of development of these organs. A segment or proglottis in which the sexual organs are developing but are not yet mature is called an *immature segment* or *immature proglottis*. A segment in which the sexual organs have matured is called a *mature segment* or *mature proglottis*. After fertilization of the eggs has been effected, both male and female sexual organs degenerate and disappear, leaving the fertilized eggs only inside the uterus or in the other organs mentioned above into which the fertilized eggs may ultimately pass. The segment is then called a *gravid segment* or *gravid proglottis* (fig. 22). In many species the gravid segment is detached from the end of the chain, which it has reached during its development and passes out of the host in the host's excreta. Some species of tapeworms thus detach gravid segments singly, as the beef tapeworm does; others detach them in short chains, as the pork tapeworm of man does. The detached gravid segments may be active and may crawl about outside the host, as those of the beef tapeworm do; or they may be inactive, as those of the pork tapeworm of man usually are. In any event, they sooner or later degenerate and disintegrate, and the eggs are thus set free. In some species (e.g. the fish tapeworm described in the next chapter), the eggs are not liberated from the final host by the detachment of gravid segments and the disintegration of these outside the host; the eggs are laid continuously into the contents of the food canal of the final host and the eggs, rather than the segments of the chain, pass out in the final host's excreta.

The Beef Tapeworm (*Taenia saginata*)

With this brief description of the general features of tapeworms in our minds, let us consider some tapeworms that are parasitic in man. The beef tapeworm, *Taenia saginata*, is one of the largest of the tapeworms and may consist of a chain of 1,000 to 2,000 segments (*proglottides*). It varies from 4 to 12 metres (13 to 39 feet) in length, but longer specimens have been found in the small intestine of man. Man is its only final host and it is found in man all over the world, although in some countries, such as Britain, it is nowadays rare. Stoll (1947) estimated that it was, in 1947, present in some 39 millions of people in the world. It may live in man for 10 years. Like the pork tapeworm, it has few intermediate hosts. Usually it is confined to intermediate hosts that belong to a single family, namely, the family Bovidae, to which the ox, buffalo, and their

117

relatives belong. Man almost always infects himself by eating
beef that contains the infective larval phase, which is a small
cyst called a bladderworm (*cysticercus*) (fig. 24), which is full
of fluid and contains a single tapeworm head.

The effects of the adult beef tapeworm on man vary in
different people. It may have so little effect on some people that
they are unaware of its presence inside them and are horrified
when the tapeworm is discovered. Other people may suffer
from abdominal pain or discomfort, increase of appetite, weakness, loss of weight, nausea, restlessness, dizziness, and a
number of other symptoms. It is said that this tapeworm may
cause, in some people, convulsions and 'fits', and these are
possibly due to poisonous substances produced by the worm.
The head of the worm may injure the walls of the small intestine and, if these injuries become infected with bacteria, ulceration of the intestinal wall may follow. It is known that some
other species of tapeworms that infect, not man, but other
hosts, do not grow so well if their hosts are kept on diets free
from the vitamins of the B group, so that possibly the beef
tapeworm removes vitamins from the food of man. It may also
remove carbohydrates from it. It does not, however, usually
cause the human host to become, as has been supposed, raven-
ous, thin, and exhausted by living 'a double life'. Its effects
are, on the whole, surprisingly benign, which is just as well,
for it can live in man for as long as ten years.

The life history of the beef tapeworm resembles that of the
pork tapeworm shown in fig. 23, except that the intermediate
host is the ox, not the pig. The chain of proglottids that is the
adult phase lives in the small intestine of man, to the wall of
which it is attached by the very small head (*scolex*), which is
pear-shaped and is only 1 to 2 mm. ($\frac{1}{25}$ to $\frac{1}{50}$ inch) in diameter. The scolex of *T. saginata* (Plate 2a) has four muscu-
lar suckers, but, unlike the scolex of the pork tapeworm of man
described below, it has no hooks. The segments of the chain of
this species have the shape shown in fig. 22. The gravid segments, which are detached singly from the chain, are 12 to 14
mm. ($\frac{1}{2}$ to $\frac{3}{4}$ inch or more) long and 4 to 7 mm. ($\frac{1}{5}$ to $\frac{3}{10}$ inch)
broad and the womb (*uterus*) in each of them, in which the

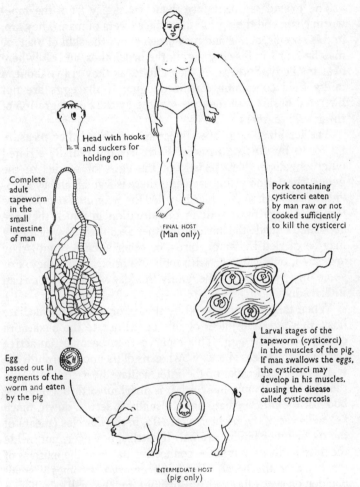

Head with hooks and suckers for holding on

Complete adult tapeworm in the small intestine of man

FINAL HOST
(Man only)

Pork containing cysticerci eaten by man raw or not cooked sufficiently to kill the cysticerci

Egg passed out in segments of the worm and eaten by the pig

Larval stages of the tapeworm (cysticerci) in the muscles of the pig. If man swallows the eggs, the cysticerci may develop in his muscles. causing the disease called cysticercosis

INTERMEDIATE HOST
(pig only)

Fig. 23. Life history of the pork tapeworm, *Taenia solium*

fertilized eggs are stored, is a straight tube running up the middle of the segment and giving off 15 to 35 lateral branches.

The gravid segments are detached singly from the tapeworm chain and they pass out in the excreta of man. They are, in this species, active and may crawl about the skin of man, or may be found in his clothing, in the bedclothes, and elsewhere near his body. Sometimes they exude, as they crawl about, a milky fluid containing fertilized eggs. If the eggs are not liberated in this way they are set free by the disintegration of the gravid segment.

The fertilized eggs are almost spherical and they measure 30 to 40 by 20 to 30 micra. Each has the radially-striated outer envelope characteristic of the eggs of species of the genus *Taenia* and inside each egg there is a small embryo provided with six hooks, which is called the *hexacanth embryo*. The fertilized eggs must wait in the situation in which they are deposited outside the host, or in other situations to which they may be carried by water, birds, or other agencies, until they are eaten, or swallowed with moisture or drink, by the ox or some other member of the family Bovidae which can act as an intermediate host.

When they are swallowed by the ox or other intermediate host, the digestive juices of this host liberate the hexacanth embryo from the egg. This embryo then becomes an active creature which tears its way by means of its hooks through the wall of the food canal of the intermediate host and gets into the blood and lymph, by which it is distributed throughout the body of the intermediate host. Usually it settles down, much as the larvae of the trichina worm do, in the muscles (meat) of the ox or other bovine animal. It settles, however, not inside the muscle fibres, but in the connective tissue of the muscles of the body or the heart. Here each embryo becomes a small bladder or cyst (fig. 24) full of fluid, on the wall of which a tapeworm head with four suckers develops. This head is at first turned outside inwards so that the four suckers on it lie on the inside of it. In this manner a larval phase, called a *cysticercus* or bladderworm, is formed. Because this is found in the muscles of the ox and other Bovidae, it is called *Cysticercus bovis*. This cysticercus is, when it is fully grown, oval and greyish-white or opalescent and it is then about 4 to 6 mm. long and about 7·5 to 10 mm. broad.

In the ox these bladderworms are found most often in the muscles of the heart and jaws, and meat-inspectors look for them in these organs; but they may also be often found in the muscles of the tongue and midriff (*diaphragm*). Less often they are found in the muscles of the neck and hind-limb or in the walls of the gullet and, indeed, in any other muscles. They do

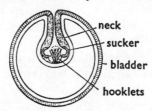

Fig. 24. Diagram of a cysticercus

not affect the health of the cattle. Cattle do not suffer even when they are, in order to test this point, so heavily infected by man that thousands of them are present.

Cysticercus bovis cannot develop further in the muscles of the intermediate host. It must wait until these muscles are eaten by the final host, man. When this happens, when, that is to say, man eats raw beef containing these bladderworms, or beef that has not been cooked, or otherwise treated in such a manner that the bladderworms are killed, the digestive juices of man dissolve the walls of the bladderworm and cause the single tapeworm head inside it to turn inside out, so that the four suckers come to lie on the outside of the tapeworm head. The head then attaches itself to the lining of the small intestine and produces the chain of segments of which the adult phase is composed.

In this life history we can note the following points:

1. One species only, namely, man, can be the final host.
2. Relatively few species can be the intermediate hosts. These are all closely-related animals, which belong to the ruminant family Bovidae. In most parts of the world the ox is virtually

the only intermediate host that conveys this parasitic animal to man.

3. This species, unlike the large intestinal fluke, includes in its life history only one period during which it must live in the world outside one or other of its hosts. This period follows the escape of its fertilized eggs from the final host. These eggs are, however, like the eggs of *Ascaris lumbricoides*, protected inside resistant envelopes. They are passive and can themselves do nothing to ensure that they are eaten by the intermediate host. For this they must rely on chance and on the habits of the final and intermediate hosts respectively.

4. There is no multiplication of the numbers of the parasitic animal inside the intermediate host. One fertilized egg can give origin only to one bladderworm and, because this contains only one tapeworm head, only a single adult tapeworm can arise from each of the fertilized eggs. Each adult tapeworm is, however, hermaphrodite, so that it is not necessary for both males and females to survive in the final host. In this respect the tapeworms resemble flukes. The adult tapeworm is not, on the other hand, a single hermaphrodite individual as the adult fluke is. It is a chain of hermaphrodite segments each of which can produce large numbers of fertilized eggs.

The Pork Tapeworm (Taenia solium)

The life history of the pork tapeworm of man, *Taenia solium*, is in most respects similar to that of the beef tapeworm just described. It is shown in fig. 23.

This species is much less common in man than the beef tapeworm is and in Britain it is nowadays never found. Stoll (1947) estimated that only about $2\frac{1}{2}$ million people in the world were infected with it at the time when he made his investigations. It is rare in the United States, but its distribution is cosmopolitan and it may turn up in man wherever control of its incidence is relaxed. Its normal intermediate host is the pig, but its larval phases can develop also in monkeys, camels, and dogs. Man, therefore, who does not normally eat monkeys, camels, or dogs, infects himself by eating the flesh of pigs that are infected with the bladderworms. To do this he must eat pigmeat that is either uncooked or has not been cooked sufficiently to kill any bladderworms in it or has not been treated with such processes as freezing, canning, or other methods of processing which normally kill these bladderworms. In countries where pork is never eaten, such as Mohammedan countries in which the eating of pork is forbidden, the pork tapeworm is correspondingly uncommon.

Another possible intermediate host of this tapeworm has not, however, been mentioned yet. This other intermediate host is man himself. If man should swallow the eggs of the pork tapeworm they may grow in his body into bladderworms, which may then have the serious effects described below.

The adult tapeworm is smaller than its relative, *Taenia saginata*. It may be 2 to 4 m. (6 to 12 ft) long, but it may reach a length of 8 m. (26 ft). It has usually only 800 to 1,000 segments and the head (*scolex*) (fig. 20) has, in addition to the four suckers, a double row of 22 to 32 hooks, which assist the tapeworm to hold on to its host.

The structure of the adult tapeworm resembles that of the beef tapeworm and it produces its fertilized eggs in the same way. The gravid segments (fig. 22B) are, however, 10 to 12 mm. long by 5 to 6 mm. broad and the uterus in them has only 7 to 12 lateral branches; they are, moreover, usually detached, not singly, but in short chains and they are not active when they have left the host. The eggs, which resemble those of the beef tapeworm, are liberated by disintegration of the segment outside the host. When they are swallowed by the intermediate host, the pig, they liberate hexacanth embryos which behave as the embryos of the beef tapeworm do. They settle in the muscles of the pig and become bladderworms which resemble those of the beef tapeworm except that the single tapeworm head inside each of them has a double row of hooks. They may be found in any of the muscles of the pig, but are most often found in the muscles of the tongue, neck, and shoulder of the pig; they may also be found in the muscles between the ribs (intercostal muscles) and in those of the abdominal region and the legs. They are usually more numerous in the pig than the bladderworm of the beef tapeworm are in the ox. They are small, whitish cysts that measure about 5 to 8 by 8 to 20 mm. and, when they are numerous, the pig-meat seems studded with small, whitish spots. It has, for this reason, been called 'measly pork'. This, however, is a bad name for it, because pork infected with the infective larvae of the trichina worm is also sometimes given this name.

Each bladderworm, if it is eaten by man while it is alive, gives origin, in the small intestine of man, to a single adult tapeworm. More than one may be present in man; and the beef and pork tapeworms may be present together in the same human being. Often, however, the presence of one tapeworm of either species prevents the establishment in the same host of another individual of the same or the other species. The presence of one tapeworm may thus confer on the person harbouring it a resistance (immunity) to infection. This resistance, however, lasts only so long as the tapeworm is present. It is, that is to say, the form of resistance called *premunity*, which lasts only so long as the particular parasite associated with it is present in the host. It can be contrasted with resistance (immunity) which persists, as the resistance of man to smallpox, for example does, long after the organism that produces it has left the host.

The effects of the pork tapeworm on the final host, man, are similar to those of the beef tapeworm described above. This species may live, it is said, for twenty-five years or longer in man. The effects of the bladderworms on the normal intermediate host, the pig, are, like those of the bladderworms of the beef tapeworm on cattle, negligible. It was, however, pointed out above that man may himself become an intermediate host. Man can, that is to say, be both the intermediate and the final host of this tapeworm. This may seem odd and is, in fact, a remarkable and unparalleled feature of this particular parasite. It is important because, when the bladderworms of the pork tapeworm develop in man – when, that is to say, man swallows, not the bladderworms, but the eggs of the tapeworm – these bladderworms cause a serious disease, called *cysticercosis*, the symptoms of which are due to the effects of the bladderworms on the human tissues in which they settle down. These effects may be especially serious when they settle, as they sometimes do, in the brain; and little can be done to cure this disease, because no drug is known that will kill the bladderworms and surgical removal of them cannot hope to remove them all when they are numerous. Because the adult pork tapeworm is parasitic only in man, human beings can become infected with the bladderworms of this tapeworm only by swallowing the eggs of the tapeworm derived from man. This happens usually when human food or drink is somehow contaminated by human faeces or with fluids, such as sewage effluents, derived from these. But man may infect himself with eggs derived from a pork tapeworm present in his own food canal. Auto-infection then occurs; and usually it occurs by contamination of the hands of the infected person with his own faeces.

The Dwarf Tapeworm (*Hymenolepis nana*)

This species is called the dwarf tapeworm, because it is the smallest tapeworm found in man. It is common also in rats and mice. Some experts think that it is identical with another species found in mice and rats which is called *Hymenolepis nana fraterna*.

Hymenolepis nana is only 25 to 40 mm. (1 to $1\frac{1}{2}$ inches) long, but it may be present in man, especially in badly-nourished children, in enormous numbers. In some of the emaciated or starved European children recovered by the Russian armies from the Germans during the Second World War thousands of these small tapeworms were found. When infections are heavy, it is often only about an inch or so long, perhaps because the competition for food among large numbers of the tapeworms causes stunting of their growth. *H. nana* is the commonest human tapeworm in the southern United States and it is also common in man in India, Egypt, and other warm countries. Stoll (1947) calculated that, at the time when he made his investigations, some 22 million people in the world were infected with this species of tapeworm. It may cause a severe illness, especially in children, the infected person suffering from abdominal pains, diarrhoea, and even convulsions and symptoms resembling those of epilepsy.

The life history of this species differs from that of nearly all other tapeworms, because it does not need an intermediate host. Its eggs, when they are laid in the food canals of man, rats, or mice, or when they are swallowed by these hosts, set free a six-hooked tapeworm embryo which makes its way, by means of its six hooks, into one of the projections (*villi*) on the surface of the lining of the small intestine. Inside this villus the embryo becomes a larval stage which corresponds to the cysticercus of the beef and pork tapeworms, but, because it develops somewhat differently and does not form a bladder of fluid, it is called a *cysticercoid* (cf. fig. 25). The cysticercoid

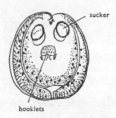

Fig. 25. The cysticercoid of the dog-tapeworm, *Dipylidium caninum*

develops inside itself a single tapeworm head and, when it is mature, it escapes into the small intestine and becomes the adult tapeworm. *H. nana* can, however, also use intermediate hosts. If its eggs are swallowed by the larvae of the fleas, *Ctenocephalides canis*, *Ctenocephalides felis*, *Xenopsylla cheopis* and *Pulex irritans* or the larvae of the grain beetle, *Tenebrio molitor*, the cysticercoid can develop in these intermediate hosts.

A species related to *H. nana* is *Hymenolepis diminuta*, which is also common in rats and mice and may also infect man, although it is much less common in man than *H. nana* is. This species uses many intermediate hosts. Among them are the young and adults of grain beetles, meal moths, earwigs, dung beetles, and fleas. Man is infected by eating cereals, dried fruits, and other foods which the insect intermediate hosts have infected with the cysticercoids of the tapeworm.

Dipylidium caninum

This species is one of the commonest tapeworms of the dog and it is the species usually found in dogs. It is also parasitic in the fox, and cat and in wild relatives of these hosts. It may also infect man, children being most often infected. In man it usually causes only relatively mild symptoms, such as intestinal discomfort and abdominal pain.

The adult tapeworm is 15 to 40 cm. (6 to 16 inches) long

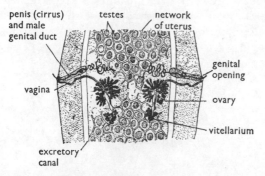

Fig. 26. A segment (proglottid) of the dog-tapeworm, *Dipylidium caninum*, showing the two sets of reproductive organs

and it may have up to 175 proglottids, each of which is shaped rather like a pumpkin seed. There is, in each segment, a double set of hermaphrodite sexual organs, so that the male and female external genital openings are also double and open on each side of each segment (fig. 26). The head (*scolex*) has four suckers and, in front of these a conical projection called the *rostellum* on which there are 30 to 150 hooks arranged in rows.

The life history utilizes fleas and the dog-louse as intermediate hosts. The eggs are set free by disintegration of gravid segments detached and passed out in the faeces. If they are swallowed by the larvae of the dog flea, (*Ctenocephalides canis*), the cat flea, (*Ctenocephalides felis*), or by the dog-louse, *Trichodectes canis*, the eggs remain little changed in these hosts, but they pass on to the adult fleas or lice and in these develop into cysticercoids similar to the cysticercoid of the dwarf tapeworm. The dog infects itself with the adult tapeworm by eating the fleas or lice, or portions of them containing the cysticercoids (fig. 25), when they cause irritation. Human beings, especially children, may accidentally ingest the cysticercoids in the same manner, when these get on to the

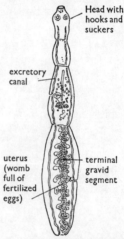

Head with hooks and suckers

excretory canal

uterus (womb full of fertilized eggs)

terminal gravid segment

Fig. 27. *Echinococcus granulosus*, the whole adult worm

fur of the dog or when they get into the mouth of the dog and it licks the hands or faces of its owners.

The species of tapeworms hitherto described, with the exception of *Taenia solium* and *Hymenolepis nana*, infect man only when they are in the adult stage, so that man is their final host. Man may also, however, be the intermediate host only of other species of tapeworms, none of which can live in him when they are adults. The most important of these species is the hydatid tapeworm, the larval phases of which are called hydatid cysts.

The Hydatid Tapeworm (*Echinococcus granulosus*)

The final hosts of this small tapeworm are the dog, the fox, the cat, and various wild relatives of the dog. The adult tapeworm (fig. 27) is small. It consists of only three or four seg-

Animals Twice Parasitic in One Life

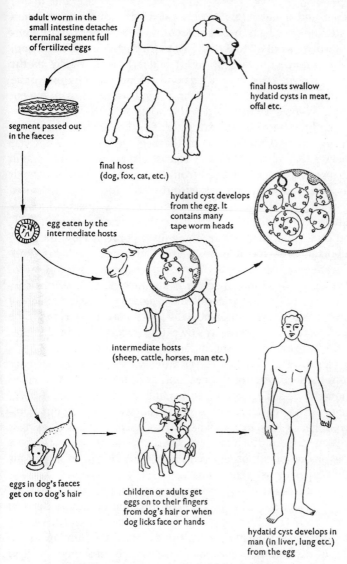

adult worm in the
small intestine detaches
terminal segment full
of fertilized eggs

final hosts swallow
hydatid cysts in meat,
offal etc.

segment passed out
in the faeces

final host
(dog, fox, cat, etc.)

hydatid cyst develops
from the egg. It
contains many
tape worm heads

egg eaten by the
intermediate hosts

intermediate hosts
(sheep, cattle, horses, man etc.)

eggs in dog's faeces
get on to dog's hair

children or adults get
eggs on to their fingers
from dog's hair or when
dog licks face or hands

hydatid cyst develops in
man (in liver, lung etc.)
from the egg

Fig. 28. Life history of *Echinococcus granulosus*

ments and a head (*scolex*) provided with four suckers and a rostellum on which there are 30 to 36 hooks. The whole adult tapeworm is only 2 to 9 mm. ($\frac{1}{12}$ to $\frac{1}{3}$ inch) long. The last segment is much the largest and it is nearly half as long as the whole worm. It is the only gravid segment at any one time. The uterus in it resembles that of the beef tapeworm, except that it has only 12 to 15 lateral branches on each side.

The life history is shown in fig. 28. The fertilized eggs in the uterus resemble those of the beef tapeworm. They are liberated by bursting of the uterus, either before the gravid segment has been detached from the whole worm, or after it has been detached and passed out of the host. The liberated eggs are swallowed by the intermediate hosts, which are numerous. Among them are man, sheep, cattle, pigs, horses, and other mammals. From the human point of view the most important intermediate hosts are man himself and his domesticated animals, because, the eggs, when they are swallowed, develop in these intermediate hosts into the type of bladderworm larval stage that is called a *hydatid cyst* and the effects of these cysts on the intermediate hosts may be serious. The final hosts infect themselves by eating parts of the dead bodies of the intermediate hosts containing the hydatid cysts.

The hydatid cyst (fig. 29B) differs in an important manner from the cysticerci of the beef and pork tapeworms described above. It is, as cysticerci also are, full of a fluid, called *hydatid fluid*, but it contains, not a single tapeworm head, but numerous heads – as many, when these cysts are large, as two million of them. Each cyst can, therefore, when it is eaten by a dog or one of the other final hosts, give origin to numerous adult tapeworms in these hosts.

What has occurred, in fact, is a multiplication, inside the intermediate host, of the number of potential adults derived from each fertilized egg. This multiplication is, therefore, comparable to the similar multiplication of the number of potential adults that occurs inside the snail intermediate host of the large intestinal fluke described above. It occurs in a different way, but it has the same result. Each egg of the parasite gives origin to a large number of potential adult parasites.

The hydatid tapeworm multiplies inside the intermediate host by a process that is shown in fig. 29B. The hexacanth embryo develops into a cyst lined by a germinal membrane which produces on its walls, not a single tapeworm head as the germinal membrane of the bladderworm (cysticercus) of the pork or beef tapeworm does, but smaller cysts, called *brood capsules*, each of which is joined to the wall of the main cyst by a stalk. Inside each brood capsule there is a germinal membrane which produces numerous separate tapeworm heads, each of

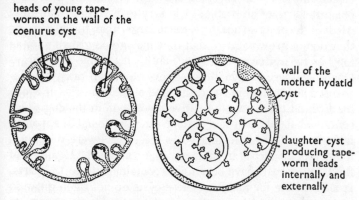

heads of young tape-
worms on the wall of the
coenurus cyst

wall of the
mother hydatid
cyst

daughter cyst
producing tape-
worm heads
internally and
externally

Fig. 29. Diagram of (A) a coenurus tapeworm cyst and (B) a hydatid cyst of *Echinococcus granulosus*

which is, like the tapeworm head in a cysticercus bladderworm, turned in on itself. The tapeworm heads thus arise inside the brood capsule rather than directly from the wall of the main cyst. Some of them may be formed directly from this wall, but most are formed inside the brood capsules. The whole cyst may also give rise to *daughter cysts*, which float in the fluid with which the mother cyst is filled; and even *granddaughter cysts* may be formed. Often the brood capsules become detached from the wall of the main cyst and fall to the bottom of it, where they may rupture and set free their tapeworm heads. They then form a deposit in the cyst, which is called *hydatid sand*.

Hydatid cysts may be found in any organ of the human body, but the liver is the commonest site of them. Next to the liver come the lungs and next to these the abdominal cavity. The cysts may also develop under the skin or in the kidney, spleen, bones, or brain. Usually the cysts are single and they grow very slowly. A month after the eggs of the tapeworm have been swallowed they are often only 1 mm. in diameter and five months later they may have become ten times this size, so that they may then be 10 mm. (half an inch) in diameter. Brood capsules are by then beginning to appear. As the cysts grow larger, more brood capsules are formed and the cyst may reach the size of an orange or it may grow larger than this. Most of the cysts do not grow much larger than this in man, or they do not grow so large; but they may go on growing for as long as twenty years and they may then become very large. One of the largest hydatid cysts ever found in man was discovered in a patient in Australia, one of the countries in which the hydatid tapeworm is relatively common in the dog. This contained about 50 quarts of fluid. Another found in a woman in Iceland, where in former years these cysts were very common, was 20 inches in diameter and contained 3½ gallons of fluid. Other cysts have been found containing 10 to 15 quarts. It is fortunate for man that these cysts do not often grow so large as this. There may, however, be several in different parts of the body of the same individual.

Usually the cysts are *unilocular*. They have, that is to say, only one cavity inside. They become, before very long, enclosed in a capsule of fibrous tissue formed by the host. This limits their growth to some extent and this is one of the host's ways of dealing with them. The cysts, however, go on growing in spite of the fibrous capsule formed by the host and, if they grow in situations in which they cannot readily expand, they may bulge out at points on their circumference where the pressure of the organs around them is less than it is elsewhere. When this happens these bulges may become nipped off, so that secondary independent cysts are formed. Another thing that may happen is that cysts growing in the firmer tissues of the body may burrow along the lines of less resistance in these tissues and the cyst then becomes, not a rounded ball, but an infiltrating mass. This may happen, for instance, when the cysts begin inside the marrow cavity of a bone; they may then fill the marrow cavity and cause erosion of the bone.

Sometimes, hydatid cysts may be found that grow, not as bladders with a single cavity, but as spongy masses without a capsule round them, in which there are several cavities containing a gelatinous material. These cysts are called *multilocular hydatid cysts*. As they go on growing they may invade the tissues surrounding them just as tumours may. This type of hydatid cyst is found in man chiefly in southern Germany, in the region of the Alps, and in Russia and Siberia as far as the Behring Sea. It has recently been shown that it results from the ingestion by man of the eggs, not of *Echinococcus granulosus*, the larval phases of which are the unilocular hydatid cysts, but those of a closely-related species, to which the name *Echinococcus multilocularis*, which is one of the names formerly given to *E. granulosus*, has recently been proposed. It is possible that *E. multilocularis* is identical with another species *Echinococcus sibiricensis*, which causes the formation of rather similar multilocular cysts in man in Siberia and the islands in the Behring Sea. A somewhat similar form of multilocular cyst, consisting of a number of small bladders that do not contain tapeworm heads, may be found in the livers of cattle; it is called *Echinococcus multilocularis veterinorum*.

Hydatid cysts are able to increase their capacity to harm man and the other intermediate hosts in which they grow by reproducing themselves in other parts of the host's body. If they become damaged, or ruptured, or if small portions of the germinal membrane which forms the tapeworm head inside them are detached, these portions can form new, independent cysts; and if they are small enough to be carried away by the blood, new cysts may arise in parts of the body distant from the original cyst. The cysts may thus be spread about the body and may appear in such vital centres as the brain and the results then are usually serious. Detached portions of the cysts that get into the blood may also block up blood vessels and have, quite apart from their ability to grow, serious effects that are due to blocking of the blood supply.

133

The chief effects of hydatid cysts are therefore (a) pressure on the tissues in which they grow, the effects of which will vary according to the situation in which the cyst lies; (b) erosion of tissues, when the cyst is of the infiltrating type; (c) blocking of blood vessels and consequent effects due to the loss of the blood supply.

It must not be thought, however, that hydatid cysts always cause serious disease. In domesticated animals they often cause little or no trouble to the animal; and probably this is true of most hydatid cysts in man. The ones that are discovered in man are those that cause symptoms which demand their removal by the surgeon who diagnoses them. Sometimes, however, they are only found when other causes demand a surgical operation. Thus the patient may be operated on for appendicitis; and during the operation hydatid cysts may be found in the abdominal cavity; or an X-ray examination, done for suspected tuberculosis or other diseases of the lung, may reveal their unsuspected presence in the lung. Many other cysts, perhaps the majority, are found only after death, when post-mortem examinations are made. Nor do the cysts, when they are found, always contain tapeworm heads. In many of them no tapeworm heads are found and these are called *sterile cysts*. The incidence of sterile cysts varies according to the intermediate host. In sheep, for instance, only eight per cent of the cysts are sterile, so that sheep are intermediate hosts in which the parasite succeeds in living successfully. It lives also fairly well in pigs, in which about twenty per cent of hydatid cysts fail to form tapeworm heads; in cattle, however, ninety per cent of them are sterile, so that these animals are not good intermediate hosts for the parasite.

The evolution of the method shown by *Echinococcus granulosus* of multiplying the number of individuals derived from each fertilized egg is perhaps indicated by the occurrence, in the life histories of some other tapeworms, of bladderworms that are intermediate between the cysticercus, which contains only a single tapeworm head, and the hydatid cyst. These species form bladderworms which contain, not brood capsules in which there are tapeworm heads, but numerous tapeworm heads which all arise from the wall of the cyst (fig. 29a). A cyst of this type is called a *coenurus* cyst.

The adult tapeworms that produce this type of bladderworm, use dogs and other carnivores as their final hosts, but usually they do not use man as an intermediate host, so that man is not usually infected with the coenurus type of cyst. This does however, occasionally occur. The tapeworm *Taenia multiceps*, for instance, the adults of which are parasitic in dogs and other carnivores, may use man as an intermediate host. Normally the coenurus cysts of these species develop in sheep, goats, or various rodents. When, however, man swallows their eggs, which he usually derives from dogs which have been infected by eating portions of the carcases of sheep or goats or rabbits infected with the cysts, the coenurus cysts may develop in man and, if they settle in certain situations, such as the brain, their effects may be serious.

In civilized communities man is infected with *Echinococcus granulosus* chiefly by swallowing the eggs of this tapeworm derived from dogs. Dogs may, for instance, contaminate human food or drink with their faeces. Foods that are especially liable to be contaminated with their eggs are salad plants, which are normally eaten uncooked. The faeces of dogs may also get on to their hair and eggs in them may be transferred to human beings when they stroke or pet the dog; or the dog may lick the eggs off its own hair and may then lick the hand or face of a human being. Children are especially liable to be infected in this way. It is possible also for dogs to deposit eggs from their mouths on to plates and dishes from which dogs are fed and, if these are used by human beings before they have been properly washed, eggs of the tapeworm remaining on them may be swallowed. In some parts of the world the fox may transmit the eggs to man, as, for example, when these animals are hunted and shot and the skin is handled when it is removed.

Infections of man with the larval phases of all these tapeworms of the dog can be prevented by keeping dogs away from the dead bodies of sheep, cattle, horses, and the other intermediate hosts; but this may be difficult or impossible in places in which these animals, and the dogs also, are allowed to roam over wide areas. Another means of control is the regular periodic treatment of dogs with drugs which will kill any adult tapeworms they may be harbouring. The efficacy of these two methods may be judged from the fact that, in Iceland, where it was estimated that, at the end of the last century, some 70,000 people kept about 20,000 dogs and a half or a third of the people had hydatid cysts, nowadays, as a result of the application of the methods of control described above, less then one per cent of the younger people in Iceland have hydatid cysts.

CHAPTER SEVEN

Animals Parasitic Three or More Times in One Life

====

In the previous chapter several species were considered, the final hosts of which infect themselves by eating the intermediate host; but in the life histories of all of them only one intermediate host was needed for the full development of the infective larva of the parasitic animal. There are, however, other species which require, not one intermediate host only, but two or more *successive* ones. The larvae of the parasitic animal develop to a certain stage only in the first intermediate host and must then pass on to a second, or even a third intermediate host to complete their development; or they develop inside the second intermediate host to the infective stage and this infective stage passes from the second intermediate host to various species which carry the infective stage about and may then infect the final host when it eats these carriers or transport hosts of the infective phase. This chapter will describe some species parasitic in man which have life histories of this kind. Man, and the other final hosts of these species, infect themselves with the adult phases of these parasitic animals by eating another animal that contains the infective phase.

The Fish Tapeworm
(*Diphyllobothrium latum* = *Dibothriocephalus latus*)

This tapeworm is called the 'fish tapeworm' because man infects himself by eating freshwater fish which contain the infective larval phase. Stoll (1947) estimated that about 10 million people in the world were infected with it at the time when he made his investigations. It is sometimes called the 'broad tapeworm', because its segments are much broader than they

137

are long. It is also called the Russian or Baltic tapeworm because it is common in man in the countries along the borders of the Baltic Sea. It also infects man in the lake districts of Switzerland and in parts of France, Bavaria, Italy, Rumania, and the Danube Basin. It has been discovered in man in Ireland. In Asia it is found in Russian Turkestan and in Palestine around Lake Tiberias. It also occurs in Japan, the Philippines and northern Manchuria. In Africa it has been found in Madagascar, Uganda, and British Bechuanaland. Immigrants from the Balkan countries have taken it to the region of the Great Lakes of North America, where it occurs especially in northern Michigan, Minnesota, and near Winnipeg. It is possible that the migrations of peoples that followed the Second World War will introduce it into other parts of Europe and elsewhere. Its distribution, however, depends, as its life history (fig. 30) shows, on the consumption by man and its other final hosts of the freshwater fishes that contain its infective phase, and infection of the final hosts can occur only if these fish are eaten raw or cooked insufficiently to kill the infective phases in them. Man therefore can control infection of himself by the simple measure of cooking these fish properly.

Infection with the fish tapeworm may cause, apart from the discomfort and other effects due simply to the bulk of this giant worm, a form of anaemia which may be severe so long as the tapeworm is present, although it usually disappears when the worm is removed and appropriate treatment of the anaemia is given.

This species of tapeworm, unlike the beef and pork tapeworms, has many final hosts. Its adult phase may be found in man, the fox, the pig, the bear, the mink, the mongoose, the seal, the sea-lion, and the walrus. Dogs can also be infected with it, but they are probably not important sources of infection, because the eggs of this tapeworm produced in them are usually incapable of further development.

The adult tapeworm, which can live in man for twenty years or more, is the largest tapeworm found in man. It may be 3 to 10 metres (9 to 33 feet) long, or, in a favourable host, rather longer than this, so that its length may be at least half the

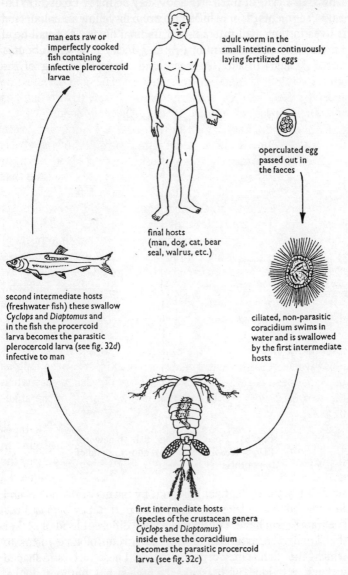

man eats raw or imperfectly cooked fish containing infective plerocercoid larvae

adult worm in the small intestine continuously laying fertilized eggs

operculated egg passed out in the faeces

final hosts (man, dog, cat, bear seal, walrus, etc.)

second intermediate hosts (freshwater fish) these swallow *Cyclops* and *Diaptomus* and in the fish the procercoid larva becomes the parasitic plerocercoid larva (see fig. 32d) infective to man

ciliated, non-parasitic coracidium swims in water and is swallowed by the first intermediate hosts

first intermediate hosts (species of the crustacean genera *Cyclops* and *Diaptomus*) inside these the coracidium becomes the parasitic procercoid larva (see fig. 32c)

Fig. 30. Life history of the fish tapeworm, *Diphyllobothrium latum*

length of a cricket pitch. Its body may be made up of 3,000 to 4,000 segments. It is whitish or greyish-yellow in colour and it lives in the small intestines of its final hosts. Its small head (*scolex*) is only 2 to 3 mm. ($\frac{1}{12}$ to $\frac{1}{8}$ inch) long and about 1 mm. ($\frac{1}{25}$ inch) broad. The head holds on to the lining of the

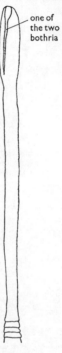

one of
the two
bothria

Fig. 31. Head of the fish tapeworm (*Diphyllobothrium latum*), showing one of the bothria

small intestine of the final host, not by means of the hooks and cup-shaped, muscular suckers that the pork tapeworm and the beef tapeworm have, but by means of a different kind of sucker that is characteristic of the different group of tapeworms to which the fish tapeworm belongs. These are slit-shaped suckers, provided with weaker muscles, but without hooks, which are called *bothria* (fig. 31) and there are, in this species, two of these, one on each side of the club-shaped or spoon-shaped head. The mature segments, found in the middle and at the lower end of the worm, are much broader than they are long. They measure 2 to 4 mm. ($\frac{1}{12}$ to $\frac{1}{6}$ inch) long by 10 to 12 mm. ($\frac{2}{5}$ to $\frac{1}{2}$ inch) and this is the reason why this species is often called the broad tapeworm.

Each segment develops, as each segment of other tapeworms also does, both male and female sexual organs, but these open to the exterior, not on the lateral edge of the segment, as the

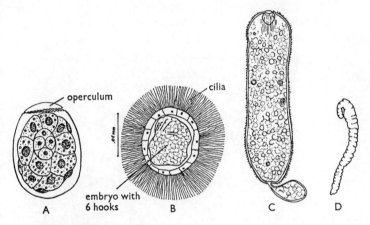

Fig. 32. (A) the egg; (B) the coracidium; (c) the procercoid larva; (D) the pleroceroid larva of the fish tapeworm, *Diphyllobothrium latum*

sexual organs of the beef and pork tapeworms do, but near to the middle of the segment (fig. 32). In each mature segment the uterus lies in the middle of the segment, but it is not a straight tube with lateral branches, as it is in the beef and pork tapeworms, but a coiled tube that looks, when it is full of eggs, rather like a dark rosette in the middle of each segment. Further, unlike the uterus of species of the genus *Taenia*, it opens to the exterior. Its external opening is in the middle of the segment, near to the openings of the male and female sexual organs (fig. 33). The broad tapeworm, moreover, does not, as the beef and pork tapeworms do, produce fertilized eggs in the

141

terminal segments only, which are cast off and discharged out of the host; it produces fertilized eggs continuously and these eggs are discharged into the contents of the food canal of the final host. The final host therefore passes out, not segments full of eggs, but the fertilized eggs themselves.

The eggs (fig. 32A) are also different from those of the beef and pork tapeworms. They are oval and measure about 60 by 42 micra. Each egg has, at its narrower end, a lid (*operculum*), similar to the operculum of the eggs of flukes.

The larval phases of the fish tapeworm are quite unlike those of the beef and pork tapeworms. Inside each egg an embryo called a *coracidium* (fig. 32B) develops in about six to ten

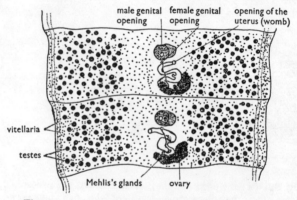

Fig. 33. A segment (proglottid) of the fish tapeworm
(*Diphyllobothrium latum*)

weeks. It is 50 to 55 micra in diameter and, like the embryos of other tapeworms, it has six small hooks. Unlike the embryos of other tapeworms, it is covered with cilia by means of which it swims, after it has left the egg, in freshwater. It can live in water for only a few hours and it dies if it is not swallowed by the first intermediate hosts.

The first intermediate hosts that this species of tapeworm can use are few. They belong to two genera only of the small, freshwater Crustacea called copepods and to only a few species of these two genera. In Europe the first intermediate hosts are *Cyclops strenuus* and *Diaptomus gracilis*; in North America three other species of the genus *Cyclops* and two others of the genus *Diaptomus* are used. Inside the bodies of these first intermediate hosts the coracidium penetrates, by means of its six hooklets, the wall of the food canal to enter the blood-space (*haemocoel*). Here it becomes an elongated larva, about 500 micra ($\frac{1}{50}$ inch) long, which is called the *procercoid larva* (fig. 32c). Usually only one or two of these procercoid larvae develop in each first intermediate host. Inside this host they must remain until the copepod is eaten by a freshwater fish in which the further development can occur.

Although so few species of copepods can act as first intermediate hosts, a number of different kinds of freshwater fishes can act as second intermediate hosts. In northern Europe the fishes involved are trout, lake trout, pike, perch, salmon, grayling, and eel; in North America the second intermediate hosts are the pike, the wall-eyed pike, the burbot, and some of their relatives. In Japan six species of Salmonidae are involved.

When these fish swallow copepods containing the procercoid larvae, the procercoids enter the muscles, connective tissue, and some of the internal organs of the fish. Here they become, in about seven to thirty days, the second larval stage, which is called the *plerocercoid* larva (fig. 32D). This is an elongate organism about 10 to 20 mm. ($\frac{2}{5}$ to $\frac{4}{5}$ inch) long and 2 to 3 mm. ($\frac{1}{12}$ to $\frac{1}{8}$ inch) broad. It may look as if its body were divided into segments, but it is not; the appearance of segmentation is caused by contractions of the body. The plerocercoid larva is the infective larva which infects the final host. It stays, protected by a cyst formed round it, in the muscles of other organs of the fish, until it reaches the food canal of the final host.

Usually human beings infect themselves by eating fish which is either not cooked at all, or is cooked so imperfectly that the plerocercoids in it are not killed. Infection may also occur when people are cleaning infected fish and the plerocercoids get on to the hands and are conveyed by them to the mouth. Plerocercoids have, however, another peculiarity. They develop chiefly in carnivorous fish and, if the fish they develop in is eaten by another fish, they can remain alive in this second

143

fish. If therefore man does not eat the fish in which they first develop, he may be infected by eating fish to which they have subsequently moved.

This ability to move from one second intermediate host to another increases this tapeworm's chances of infecting its final hosts and compensates no doubt, for the handicap of being able to use only a few first intermediate hosts. It is excelled, as a means of reaching the final hosts, by tapeworms of the genus *Spirometra*, which are related to species of the genus *Diphyllobothrium*. The plerocercoid larvae of species of the genus *Spirometra* were given the generic name *Sparganum* before it was known that they are, not adult tapeworms, but the plerocercoid larvae of tapeworms that become adult in dogs, cats, and other mammalian hosts. They are nowadays often called *spargana*. Normally these plerocercoids (spargana) of species of the genus *Spirometra* develop in frogs, snakes, birds or mammals, which swallow the first intermediate hosts, which are usually species of the genus *Cyclops*; but man may also swallow these copepods and, if he does so, the plerocercoids (spargana) may develop in him and may cause disease. Man is then, of course, acting, as freshwater fish do for the fish-tapeworm, as a second intermediate host of some species of the genus *Spirometra*. But man can infect himself with these plerocercoids (spargana), not only by swallowing the first intermediate hosts, but also in another way. Being plerocercoids, these spargana can pass, as the plerocercoids of the fish tapeworm can, from one second intermediate host to another. They can, moreover, do this, not only when one second intermediate host eats another second intermediate host, but also when the flesh of one second intermediate host comes into contact with the flesh of another. In the Far East, for example, a method of treating inflamed eyes or injuries and wounds is to apply to the injury a poultice made of fresh frog's flesh and, when plerocercoids (spargana) are present in the flesh of the frog used, these may pass directly from the frog to the human tissues to which the frog's flesh has been applied. Infection with the spargana is then added to the existing injury. The flesh of the frog may contain, for instance, plerocercoids of a tapeworm called *Spirometra erinacei,* the final hosts of which are dogs, cats, and their wild relatives. Infection of man with its plerocercoids (sparganosis), acquired in the manner just described, occurs in China, Japan, Indo-China, the Malay Archipelago, Africa, Australia, British Guiana, and Puerto Rico.

Another species of tapeworm whose plerocercoids (spargana) may be found in man is *Spirometra mansonoides,* the final hosts of which are cats and wild cats in North America. Serious symptoms may result when these plerocercoids develop in man and migrate about his body. The plerocercoid larva of another tapeworm the adult form of which is not known, is called *Sparganum proliferum,* because it produces irregular lateral processes, which bud off new plerocercoid larvae, so that enormous numbers of plerocercoid larvae may develop thus asexually from a single larva. These may wander about in the body and cause serious disease. They are found in man chiefly in Japan, but one human infection with them has been found in North America. Possibly the asexual multiplication of the plerocercoids of this species which occurs in man is an abnormal process that occurs in man because he is not one of the normal second intermediate hosts. It is well known that parasitic animals of all kinds, whether their life histories are direct or indirect, behave abnormally, and may produce more serious effects, in the bodies of hosts that are not the ones that normally they use.

FLUKES WITH TWO SUCCESSIVE INTERMEDIATE HOSTS

The life history of the broad tapeworm may be compared with the life histories of five species of flukes (Trematoda) which cause human disease and use two successive intermediate hosts. These species are:

1. The Chinese or Oriental Liver Fluke, *Opisthorchis (Clonorchis) sinensis.*
2. The cat liver fluke, *Opisthorchis felineus.*

These two species belong to the family of flukes called

the Opisthorchiidae and they use snails as their first, and fishes as their second, intermediate hosts. Man and the other final hosts infect themselves by eating fish infected with the cercariae when the fish are eaten raw or have not been cooked sufficiently to kill the cercariae in them.

3. *Heterophyes heterophyes.*
4. *Metagonimus yokogawai.*

These two species belong to the family of flukes called the Heterophyidae. They also use snails as their first, and fishes as their second intermediate hosts and man and the

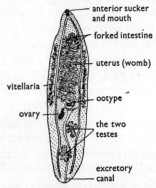

anterior sucker
and mouth

forked intestine

uterus (womb)

vitellaria

ootype

ovary

the two
testes

excretory
canal

Fig. 34. The oriental liver fluke of man
(*Opisthorchis* (*Clonorchis*) *sinensis*). Hermaphrodite adult

final (definitive) hosts infect themselves by eating fish infected with the cercariae either raw or insufficiently cooked.

5. The Oriental Lung Fluke, *Paragonimus westermanii*, which belongs to the family of flukes called the Troglotrematidae. This species uses snails as its first intermediate hosts and crayfish or crabs as its second intermediate hosts and man and the other final hosts infect themselves by eating cray-fish or crabs either raw or insufficiently cooked.

The Chinese or Oriental Liver Fluke (*Opisthorchis sinensis*)

The adult of this species is shown in fig. 34 and its life history in fig. 35. It is still often known by its former name,

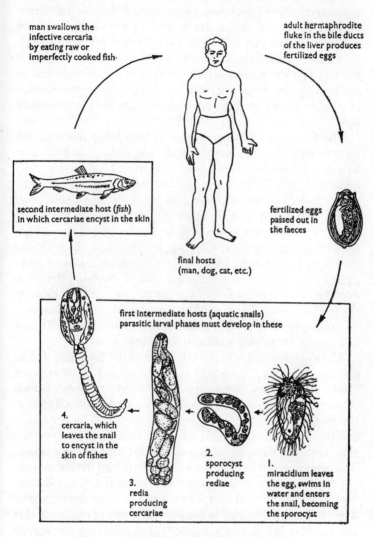

man swallows the
infective cercaria
by eating raw or
imperfectly cooked fish

adult hermaphrodite
fluke in the bile ducts
of the liver produces
fertilized eggs

second intermediate host (*fish*)
in which cercariae encyst in the skin

fertilized eggs
passed out in
the faeces

final hosts
(man, dog, cat, etc.)

first intermediate hosts (aquatic snails)
parasitic larval phases must develop in these

4.
cercaria, which
leaves the snail
to encyst in the
skin of fishes

3.
redia
producing
cercariae

2.
sporocyst
producing
rediae

1.
miracidium leaves
the egg, swims in
water and enters
the snail, becoming
the sporocyst

Fig. 35. Life history of the oriental liver fluke,
Opisthorchis sinensis

Clonorchis sinensis. Its life history resembles that of the fish tapeworm, *Diphyllobothrium latum*, except that its first intermediate hosts are snails. Its second intermediate hosts are numerous fishes that belong to the carp family (Cyprinidae). A further difference between these two life histories is the fact that the second intermediate host is infected, not by swallowing the first intermediate host, but by penetration of its skin by the cercaria derived from the first intermediate host.

The final hosts of this species include man, the dog, the cat and wild cat, the marten, mink, and badger, and the pig. The adult fluke infects the liver of man and these other final hosts in Japan, China, Formosa, and Indo-China; it is especially prevalent in Japan, Korea, and South-eastern China. Stoll (1947) estimated that about 19 million people in the world were infected with it at the time when he made his investigations. It is a flattened and elongate, greyish fluke about 11·5 to 20·1 mm. ($\frac{1}{2}$ to $\frac{4}{5}$ inch) long and 2·8 to 4·6 mm. (about $\frac{1}{10}$ to $\frac{2}{10}$ inch) broad. It lives in the distal ends of the tubes that conduct the bile out of the liver (bile ducts), especially in those of the left lobe of the liver; rarely it may invade the gall bladder. In this situation it is often coloured brown by the bile. It may live in man for as long as fifteen to twenty years.

The eggs are laid into the bile ducts of the final host. In the cat this fluke may lay 2,500 eggs a day, and in other hosts about 1,000 a day. Each egg has a light, yellowish-brown colour and it measures on an average 29 by 16 micra. It has at the narrower end, the lid (*operculum*) that all fluke eggs have and the shell projects a little all round this. Inside the egg the first larva, the miracidium, has developed when the egg is laid. The eggs pass out of the liver with the bile into the intestine of the final host and are voided with the faeces. They do not hatch outside the final host, as the eggs of other flukes do, but hatch only when the egg is swallowed by one of the snails that are the first intermediate hosts. These snails are operculate aquatic snails belonging to several genera, so that this fluke has several first intermediate hosts. Inside the snail, the egg hatches in the food canal and makes its way into the lymph spaces of this host, in which it becomes the sporocyst. The sporocyst produces rediae, each of which produces 6 to 8 cercariae and these make their way out of the snail into the water in which it lives. Each cercaria is a young fluke. It has an ellipsoid body that measures 130 to 170 by 60 to 80 micra ($\frac{1}{200}$ to $\frac{1}{147}$ by about $\frac{1}{400}$ to $\frac{1}{300}$ inch) and a long tail, about 330 to 380 micra long.

The cercaria lives only 24 to 48 hours and dies inless it meets and penetrates into the skin of one of the second intermediate hosts. There are about forty species of these second intermediate hosts and they are all freshwater fishes belonging to the carp family, which are often eaten raw or imperfectly cooked by man. Some of them are cultivated in artificial ponds as food. When the cercaria comes into contact with one of them it bores its way in beneath the scales and there becomes enclosed in a cyst, which measures about 138 by 115 micra (about $\frac{1}{180}$ by $\frac{1}{217}$ inch). Inside this cyst the cercaria must remain until one of the final hosts eats the freshwater fish either raw or imperfectly cooked.

The adult phase of this species is thus, as the broad tapeworm also is, a parasite of fish-eating mammals, and its life history resembles that of the broad tapeworm, except that it uses snails as its first intermediate hosts and uses a different method of getting into the second intermediate hosts. It does not, that is to say, wait, as the broad tapeworm does, inside the protection of the body of the first intermediate host until this is swallowed by the second intermediate host, but actively makes its way out of the first intermediate host to brave the world outside this host until it meets, and penetrates into, the second intermediate host.

The effects of this fluke upon man may, if the flukes are not numerous, be no more than localized inflammation of the bile ducts, especially those of the left lobe of the liver. Often, however, the flukes are very numerous; as many as 21,000 of them have been found after death in man. When they are numerous the flukes cause serious disease. In the liver they irritate the bile ducts and cause overgrowth of the cells lining these ducts and eventually the ducts may become thickened or dilated and there may be inflammation in and around them, accompanied by fibrosis, enlargement of the liver, and the formation of new bile ducts. The disease develops slowly and is chronic. The final results of the enlargement of, and other effects on, the liver include diarrhoea, oedema, ascites, and ultimate death.

The Cat Liver Fluke (*Opisthorchis felineus*)

This relative of the Chinese liver-fluke was first found in the cat, but it also uses man, the dog, the fox, the wolverine, and the seal as its final hosts. In man it is found in Central and Eastern Europe, East Prussia, Poland, the Dnieper and Donetz Basins, and in Siberia and in India, China, and Japan, and the Philippine Islands. Stoll (1947) estimated that about one million people in the world were infected with this species at the time when he made his investigations, most of them being in Eastern Europe and Russia. *O. felineus* is a lancet-shaped, small fluke, 7 to 12 mm. ($\frac{3}{10}$ to $\frac{1}{2}$ inch) long, and 2 to 3 mm. (about $\frac{1}{10}$ inch) broad. The adult lives in the bile ducts of the final hosts. The eggs resemble those of the Chinese liver fluke and are about the same size. The life history also resembles that of the Chinese liver fluke, but the intermediate hosts are few; there are one or two species of snails belonging to the genus *Bithynia* (*Bulimus*) only. After developing in these snails the cercariae penetrate into various cyprinoid freshwater fishes and the final hosts infect themselves by eating these fishes either raw or not cooked sufficiently to kill the cercariae in them.

In man this fluke does not usually disturb the functions of the liver, but continued infections may establish up to a thousand or so of the adult flukes in the bile ducts, and then enlargement of the liver, congestion of it with blood, jaundice, liver fibrosis, and gallstones may result.

Heterophyes heterophyes

This small fluke (fig. 36) is only 1 to 1·7 mm. ($\frac{1}{25}$ to $\frac{1}{14}$ inch) long and 0·3 to 0·4 mm. (about $\frac{1}{80}$ to $\frac{1}{60}$ inch) broad. It belongs, as *Metagonimus yokogawai* next to be described also does, to the family of flukes called the Heterophyidae. A feature of the anatomy of flukes belonging to this family is that there is, alongside the ventral sucker, near the middle of the body, another sucker inside which the male and female genital openings lie, called the genital sucker. All members of the family Heterophyidae use snails as their first, and fishes as their second, intermediate hosts.

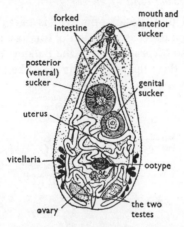

Fig. 36. *Heterophyes heterophyes.* Hermaphrodite adult

The final hosts of *Heterophyes heterophyes* are man, the dog, the cat, the fox, and other fish-eating mammals. The adult lives in the small intestine of the final host. It is common in man in the Nile Delta and in Japan, China, Formosa, and the Philippine Islands. Its life history resembles that of *M. yokogawai* and also that of the Chinese liver fluke. The eggs are minute and ovoid; they measure only 28 to 30 micra by 15 to 17 micra. The first intermediate host in Egypt is the snail *Pirenella conica* and in Japan a snail that lives in brackish water, called *Cerithidia cingulata*. The cercaria which develops in these snails resembles that of *Metagonimus yokogawai*. The second intermediate hosts are the grey mullet (*Mugil cephalus*) and related fish. The final hosts infect themselves by eating these fish either raw or insufficiently cooked.

This fluke usually causes only a mild inflammation of the small intestine of man. It may, however, burrow into the lining of the small intestine and it is stated that its eggs may then get into the blood or lymph of the final host and be carried to the heart or brain, with the result that heart failure or cerebral haemorrhage may occur.

Metagonimus yokogawai

The adult of this species (fig. 37) is parasitic in man in China, Japan, and the coastal region of Russia adjacent to these countries. It also occurs in man in the Balkan area of Europe. It also uses the dog, the cat, the pig, and the pelican as final

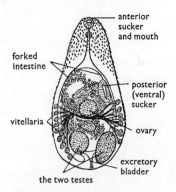

Fig. 37. *Metagonimus yokogawai*. Hermaphrodite adult

hosts. It is a small fluke, 1 to 1·25 mm. (about $\frac{1}{20}$ inch) long and 0·4 to 0·75 mm. ($\frac{1}{60}$ to $\frac{1}{33}$ inch) broad, and beside its ventral sucker there is a muscular ring round a depression in which the male and female sexual openings lie.

The life history and the eggs are similar to those of the Chinese liver fluke (fig. 35) and are about the same size as those of *Heterophyes heterophyes*. The first intermediate host is a snail belonging to the genus *Melania*. In this snail the sporocyst and two generations of rediae develop. The cercaria produced in the snail has a tail provided with fins. It enters the skin of fishes used as food by man, among which the trout

Plecoglossus altivelis plays an important part in infecting man. The final hosts infect themselves by eating these fishes either raw or insufficiently cooked.

This species of fluke burrows into the lining of the small intestine and causes irritation, one result of which is diarrhoea. The eggs, like those of *Heterophyes heterophyes*, may get into the blood and lymph of the final host and may then be carried to the heart, brain, and other organs, where they may cause irritation and tissue changes with results similar to those caused by the eggs of *Heterophyes heterophyes* described above.

The Oriental Lung Fluke (Paragonimus westermanii)

The life history of this species is shown in fig. 38. It is similar to the history of the Oriental liver fluke, except that, although the first intermediate hosts are aquatic snails, the second intermediate hosts are, not fish, but freshwater crayfishes and crabs, which are eaten raw by man. The final hosts of the adult flukes are numerous. They include, in addition to man, the dog, fox, wolf, cat, wild cat, tiger, mountain lion, the weasel, the marten, mink, badger, the rat and musk-rat, the oppossum, and the goat and pig. The fluke has a wider geographical distribution than the Oriental liver fluke has, but its distribution is usually localized and perhaps for this reason it infects relatively few people. Stoll (1947) estimated that only about three million people in the world were infected with it at the time when he made his investigations. In man it is found in Japan, Korea, China, Formosa, Indo-china and the Philippines, in Siam and Malaya, in Assam and India, and in New Guinea and adjacent islands. In South America it occurs in Brazil, Ecuador, Peru, and Venezuela, and in Africa five cases have been recorded from Nigeria and the Belgian Congo. In North America only one case of infection of man is known. Probably man protects himself by the cooking methods used; but in other mammals the fluke is found in Minnesota, Michigan, Wisconsin, Ohio, New York, Mississippi, Kentucky, South Carolina, and California; it also occurs in Northern Canada.

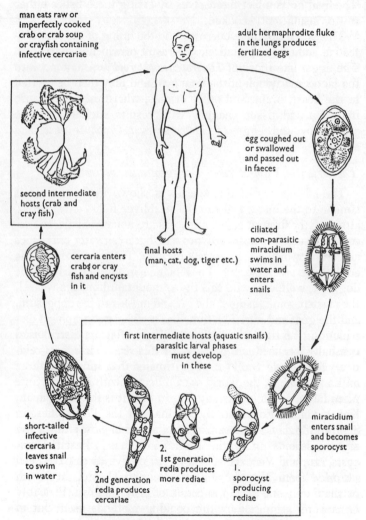

man eats raw or imperfectly cooked crab or crab soup or crayfish containing infective cercariae

adult hermaphrodite fluke in the lungs produces fertilized eggs

egg coughed out or swallowed and passed out in faeces

second intermediate hosts (crab and cray fish)

cercaria enters crabs or cray fish and encysts in it

final hosts (man, cat, dog, tiger etc.)

ciliated non-parasitic miracidium swims in water and enters snails

first intermediate hosts (aquatic snails) parasitic larval phases must develop in these

miracidium enters snail and becomes sporocyst

4. short-tailed infective cercaria leaves snail to swim in water

3. 2nd generation redia produces cercariae

2. 1st generation redia produces more rediae

1. sporocyst producing rediae

Fig. 38. Life history of the oriental lung fluke of man (*Paragonimus westermanii*)

The adult fluke (fig. 39) is reddish-brown and its size and shape vary because it is constantly expanding and contracting, so that the size of the living fluke cannot be accurately stated. When it has been preserved the fluke measures about 0·8 to 1·6 cm. long ($\frac{3}{10}$ to $\frac{6}{10}$ inch) by 0·4 to 0·8 cm. broad, and its skin, like that of many other flukes, is covered with spines. It lives inside reddish-brown nodules in the lungs of the final hosts. These nodules contain one or more cystic cavities inside

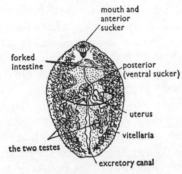

Fig. 39. The oriental lung fluke of man (*Paragonimus westermanii*). Hermaphrodite adult

which the flukes live and lay their eggs. Usually there is only one fluke in each cyst. These cysts containing flukes may, however, be found in other parts of the body of the final host, such as the muscle of the food canal, the abdominal cavity, the pleural spaces round the lungs, the liver, the muscles, and skin and also in the brain.

The eggs of this fluke, which are oval and yellowish-brown and measure 85 by 53 micra, escape from the cysts when the cysts rupture. Cysts in the lungs rupture into the air tubes (bronchi) and the eggs then either leave the host in its sputum or they are swallowed and pass out in the faeces of the host. Outside the host a miracidium develops in each egg. In this respect, therefore, the Oriental lung fluke differs from the Oriental live fluke, the miracidium of which is already formed when the egg is laid.

When it is mature the miracidium escapes through the

155

opercular lid of the egg and swims by means of its cilia. It can live only about a day and dies if it does not meet with one of the aquatic snails that can act as first intermediate hosts. When it meets one of these snails, the miracidium bores its way through the head or mantle of the snail and reaches the lymph spaces, in which it becomes the sporocyst, which is an elongate, saccular structure about 400 micra long and 160 micra broad. Each sporocyst produces a first generation of 20 to 26 rediae and these live near the digestive gland or the food canal of the snail. Some sixty days later they produce a second generation of rediae and these produce the cercariae. Each cercaria has an ellipsoid body which measures 225 by 80 micra. Its tail, however, is very short; it is only about $\frac{1}{12}$ of the length of the body (19 micra).

The cercariae make their way out of the snail and swim in the water. They die within forty-eight hours unless they meet with one of the crabs or crayfish which are the second intermediate hosts. When this happens they bore in between the chitinous plates with which the bodies of these animals are covered and make their way to various organs of these hosts, in which they encyst. In crabs and crayfish these cysts, which measure 245 to 450 micra in diameter, may be found in the gills, the liver, the muscles of the limbs, and in other organs. Often they are numerous around the heart. Here the cercariae remain until the crab or crayfish is eaten by one of the final hosts. When this happens the digestive juices of the stomach dissolve away the tissues of the second intermediate host in which the cercariae are embedded and the digestive ferments of the duodenum liberate the cercariae from the cyst. The cercariae then make their way through the walls of the food canal into the abdominal cavity, from which they penetrate the midriff (diaphragm) to reach the lungs in which they become enclosed in cysts. They may be found in the cysts twenty days after the second intermediate host was eaten.

The effects of the Oriental lung fluke on man vary to some extent according to where the flukes settle down in the human body, but the disease they cause develops slowly and is chronic. There may be a generalized type of disease, the symptoms of which are slight fever, enlargement of the lymphatic glands, and pains resembling those caused by rheumatism. The flukes in the lungs cause symptoms which may resemble those of tuberculosis. A cough develops, with pains in the chest and blood-stained sputum containing pus may be brought up, or cysts containing the flukes may burst into the air-tubes and their contents may be coughed up. Actual bleeding from the lungs may occur. Another form of the disease may occur when the eggs of the flukes penetrate into the walls of the intestine. Intestinal ulceration may then develop, with perhaps abdominal pain, diarrhoea, and the passage of blood and mucus in the faeces. Yet another type of the disease is caused when the flukes get into the brain and cause cerebral symptoms. These may resemble the symptoms of Jacksonian epilepsy and various paralyses may occur.

CHAPTER EIGHT

The Malarial Parasites

THESE parasites are single-celled Protozoa and they all belong to the single genus *Plasmodium*. Four species of them occur in the blood and other organs of man and cause the serious disease called malaria. Other species are found in the blood and other organs of monkeys, bats, rodents, buffalo, antelope, and many birds, among which are the English sparrow (*Passer domesticus*), the robin, the starling, the domestic fowl, and certain kinds of pheasants and ducks. All the species, whether they are parasitic in man or in birds, are, during the part of the life history that occurs in mammals or birds, intracellular parasites, which live inside the red cells of the blood, or inside the cells of the liver or other organs. Inside these cells the malarial parasites multiply their numbers by asexual multiple division. When this multiplication ceases, male and female gametocytes appear in the blood and these are taken up by the mosquito when it sucks the blood of the vertebrate host. Inside the body of the mosquito the malarial parasites undergo a sexual process which produces an infective phase and this infective phase is transmitted back into the blood of the vertebrate host when the mosquito again sucks blood.

The life histories of all the malarial parasites are therefore indirect. The mosquitoes are the final hosts and the vertebrate hosts (man and birds) are the intermediate hosts. The parasites remain, throughout the whole of their life histories, inside either the intermediate or the final host and never enter the world outside these hosts. They could not survive in this outer world if they entered it. They may be compared, in this respect, to the trichina worm described in chapter 4, but the life history of this worm is, it will be remembered, direct, not indirect.

The species of malarial parasites which infect birds cannot

infect man. They are transmitted to birds by mosquitoes belonging to the genera *Aedes*, *Culex*, and *Theobaldia*, which do not transmit the human malarial parasites. The species that occur in man are transmitted to him only by mosquitoes belonging to the genus *Anopheles* and only by certain species of this genus. The parasites are, moreover, transmitted only by the females of this species of the genus *Anopheles*, because the females only suck blood; the males feed on the juices of fruits and other liquids. The human malarial parasites are, therefore, good examples of species of parasitic animals which are adapted to life in relatively few hosts. They are restricted to the use of the female mosquitoes only of certain species only of single genus *Anopheles* as their final hosts; and their only intermediate host, with the exception of certain monkeys, is man.

The Human Malarial Parasites

Four species of the genus *Plasmodium* may be found in man. The names given to these four species are: *Plasmodium vivax*, which causes benign tertian malaria; *Plasmodium falciparum*, which causes malignant or aestivo-autumnal malaria; *Plasmodium malariae*, which causes quartan malaria; and *Plasmodium ovale*, which causes a form of tertian malaria. The meaning of these terms given to the various forms of malaria will be explained after the life histories of the malarial parasites have been described.

The life histories of all the species that occur in man are similar and the life history of *Plasmodium vivax* (fig. 40) may be taken as a type of them all. It looks a complicated affair, but it is, in fact, simply a life history divided into two phases – an asexual phase of multiplication in the cells of the liver and blood of man and a sexual phase inside the body of the mosquito. Let us take the former first.

The asexual phase in the body of man begins with the infective phase produced in the body of the mosquito. This is a minute spindle-shaped cell, called a *sporozoite*, which is injected by the mosquito into the blood of man when the mosquito sucks human blood. The sporozoites, thousands of which

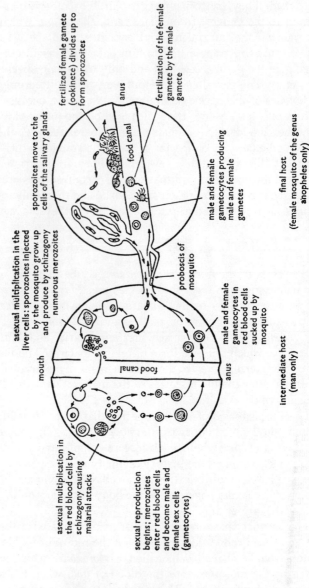

Fig. 40. Life history of a human malarial parasite, *Plasmodium vivax*

asexual multiplication in the liver cells: sporozoites injected by the mosquito grow up and produce by schizogony numerous merozoites

fertilized female gamete (ookinete) divides up to form sporozoites

sporozoites move to the cells of the salivary glands

anus

food canal

fertilization of the female gamete by the male gamete

male and female gametocytes producing male and female gametes

proboscis of mosquito

mouth

food canal

anus

asexual multiplication in the red blood cells by schizogony causing malarial attacks

sexual reproduction begins; merozoites enter red blood cells and become male and female sex cells (gametocytes)

male and female gametocytes in red blood cells sucked up by mosquito

intermediate host (man only)

final host (female mosquito of the genus anopheles only)

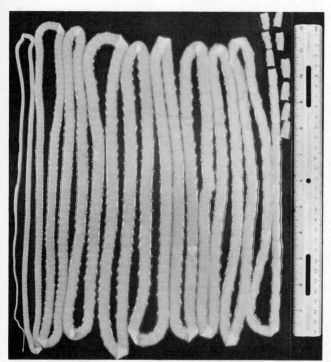

(a) *Fasciola hepatica*, the common liver fluke of sheep, cattle, man, etc. An example of a hermaphrodite Trematode.

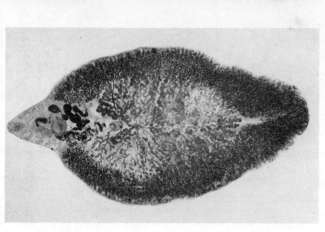
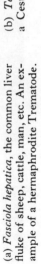

(b) *Taenia saginata*, the beef tapeworm of man. An example of a Cestode worm.

1

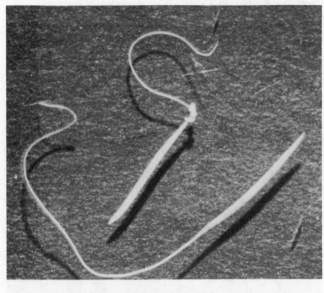

(b) *Trichuris trichiura*, a whipworm. An example of a roundworm (Nematoda).

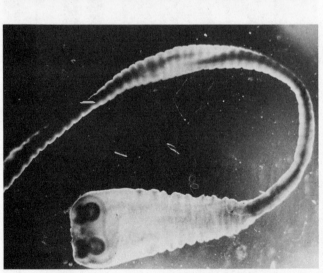

(a) Head of *Taenia saginata*, the beef tapeworm of man, showing the four suckers.

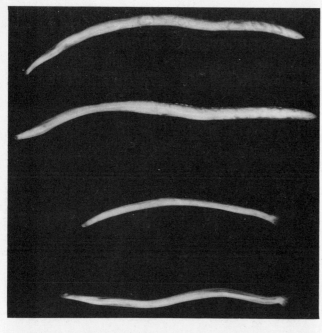

(a) *Enterobius vermicularis*, the human threadworm (seatworm). Adult females. Roundworms (Nematoda).

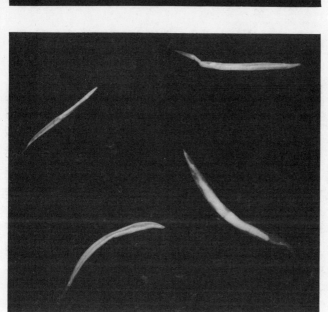

(b) Human Hookworms. *Left*, two adult males; *right*, two adult females. Roundworms (Nematoda).

3

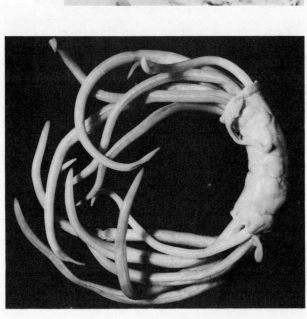

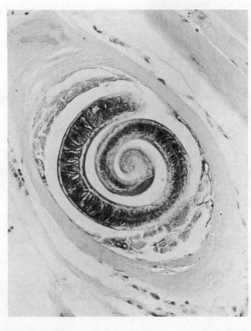

(a) *Ascaris lumbricoides*, the large roundworm (Nematoda) parasitic in man and the pig. Adults blocking up the piece of the small intestine shown.

(b) Larva of the trichina worm, *Trichinella spiralis*, coiled in its cyst in the muscle of its host.

4

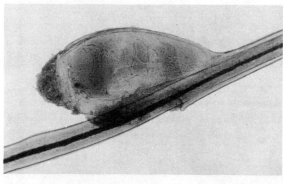

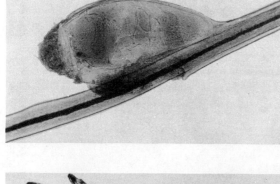

(a) The human head louse, *Pediculus humanus* var. *capitis*, a wingless insect adapted for life on the skin of its host. Note the claws for holding on and the body flattened from above downwards.

(b) Egg (nit) of the human head louse, attached to a human hair.

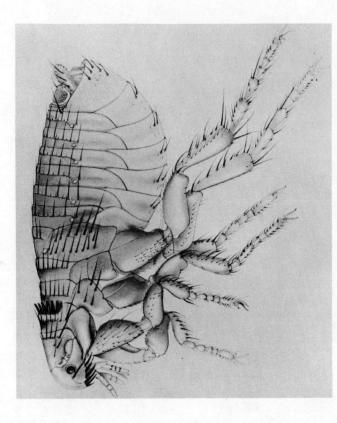

The Cat-Flea, *Ctenocephalides felis felis*, a wingless insect with large legs for leaping and a laterally-flattened body.

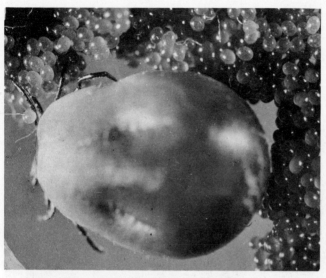

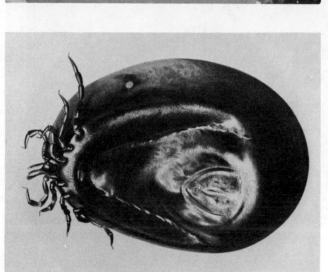

Left, Ixodes ricinus, the common tick of sheep and cattle, ventral view. An example of a hard tick. Right, the female Ixodes ricinus laying eggs.

7

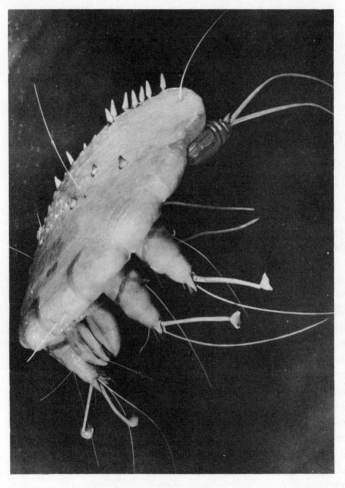

Sarcoptes scabiei, the cause of human scabies and sarcoptic mange of animals.

may be injected into the blood of man, are carried by the blood to the liver of man and there they enter the cells of the liver and feed on the substance of these. When their growth is completed, the nucleus of each of them divides into many daughter-nuclei and the body then divides into a number of daughter individuals which corresponds to the number of nuclei pr oduced.

This kind of division, the division, that is to say, of the whole body of the parasite into a number of individuals produced simultaneously, is called *multiple division* or *schizogony*, to distinguish it from division of the body into two parts only, which is called *binary* fission. The parent individual which undergoes schizogony is called a *schizont*.

Multiple division (*schizogony*) occurs during the life histories of other kinds of parasitic Protozoa and it greatly increases the number of individual parasites. The products of it, the small individuals, that is to say, into which the parent parasite divides, are called *merozoites*. Each individual of *Plasmodium falciparum* may produce, in about six days, some 40,000 merozoites in the liver of man, but other species produce much smaller numbers of them. *P. vivax*, for example, produces only about 1,000.

The merozoites produced in this manner in the liver pass into the blood and there attack the red blood cells, inside which the process of multiplication by multiple division (schizogony) is repeated several times. The merozoite, after it has entered a red blood cell, becomes at first a phase called the *signet-ring stage*, a name which was given to this stage because, when it is coloured by the red and blue aniline dyes used to show up these parasites inside the red blood cells, the nucleus of the parasite appears as a small red dot in a ring of blue cytoplasm, the interior of the parasite being uncoloured because it is a vacuole full of fluid which does not take up the dye. Later the parasite grows and becomes a small amoeba which eventually almost fills the red blood cell on which it feeds. When it is full-grown it repeats, inside the red blood cell, the process of multiple division (schizogony) that occurred in the cells of the liver. It splits up into a number of merozoites, each of which is an independent individual. *Plasmodium vivax* forms in this manner 12 to 24 merozoites; *P. ovale* forms 8 of them; *P. malariae* forms 6 to 10 and *P. falciparum* 8 to 24, the average number being 16. The number of individuals (*merozoites*) produced by multiple division inside the red blood cells is therefore much smaller than the number of them produced in the liver. It is, however, repeated several times.

During its life inside the red blood cell, each individual malarial parasite damages its host-cell and eventually destroys it. When the schizogony of the parasite is complete, the host-cell bursts and the merozoites formed by the multiple division are set free into the blood. They then attack healthy red blood cells and, feeding on these, repeat the process of schizogony, so that more merozoites are produced and these may again repeat this process of multiplication. In this manner thousands, and sometimes millions, of malarial parasites may be produced in the blood. The total number of parasites that may be present in the whole of the blood in the body is further discussed in chapter 11.

When the impulse to multiply asexually by schizogony is exhausted, the merozoites grow up, not into individuals (schizonts) which again divide up, but into male and female individuals, called *gametocytes*, which cannot develop further in the blood of man. To develop further they must enter the body of the mosquito which is the final host. When the mosquito sucks up human blood containing the gametocytes, any other phases of the malarial parasite that may be present in the blood are digested in the mosquito's food canal. The gametocytes, however, survive. They produce in the midgut (stomach) of the female anopheline mosquito, the male and female sex-cells (gametes). The nucleus of the female gametocyte undergoes a process akin to the reduction of the number of chromosomes in the formation of the unfertilized egg of higher animals and the female gametocyte is then a female gamete ready to be fertilized. The nucleus of the male gametocyte divides up into several pieces, each of which goes into one of several long, thin, protoplasmic processes that appear as the surface of the male gametocyte. Each of these processes becomes a male gamete, equivalent to a mammalian spermatozoon. The male gametes, each of which is 20 to 25 micra long, then break away from the male gametocyte and swim away to fertilize the female gametes. The fertilized female gamete is then called the *zygote*. It corresponds to the fertilized egg of the higher animals. Its fertilization usually occurs twenty minutes to two hours after the gametocytes have been taken in by the mosquito.

Soon after its fertilization the zygote becomes a motile organism about 18 to 24 micra long, which is now called the *ookinete*. The ookinete glides along in the contents of the mosquito's midgut and eventually penetrates through the wall of the midgut to settle down just under the thin, elastic membrane that separates the midgut from the blood-space (*haemocoel*) around it. Here the ookinete becomes surrounded by a membrane formed partly by the food canal of the mosquito and partly by itself and becomes, about 48 hours after the gametocytes were taken in, the *oocyst*. The oocysts grow till they are 40 to 80 micra in diameter and they can be seen on the outside of the midgut as transparent, rounded structures. Inside them the nucleus divides up repeatedly and the cytoplasm divides up into minute, spindle-shaped individuals, called *sporozoites*. Each sporozoite contains one of the products of the division of the nucleus of the zygote. The oocyst then bursts into the blood-space outside the midgut and the sporozoites, liberated into the blood in this space, find their way to the salivary glands of the mosquito. Here they remain until they are injected back into man when the mosquito again sucks human blood.

The time required for the entire sexual development in the mosquito varies according to the species of malarial parasite and the mosquito concerned and also according to the temperature outside the mosquito's body. The sexual cycle of *P. vivax* takes about 16 days when the outside temperature is 20° C and 17 to 18 days when it is 23 to 28° C. The sexual development of *P. ovale* takes about 16 days when the external temperature is 25° C. The sexual cycle of *P. falciparum* takes about 22 days when the external temperature is 20° C, about 17 to 18 days when it is 23 to 28° C and about 10 to 11 days when it is 30° C. The sexual development of *P. malariae* takes about 30 to 35 days when the external temperature is 20° C and about 28 days when it is 23 to 28° C. Colder weather therefore slows up the sexual development and this is, as we shall learn later in this book, one of the reasons why malarial parasites often do not succeed in producing sporozoites in the relatively cold summer temperatures in England and then cannot, for this reason, infect man in this country.

The number of sporozoites produced by this process of multiplication inside the oocyst is prodigious. It depends partly on the number of oocysts that succeed in developing. Normally only a small percentage of the gametocytes ingested by the mosquito succeed in producing sporozoites. There may be, however, 50 oocysts on the wall of the midgut of the mosquito and each may produce 10,000 sporozoites, so that theoretically the number of sporozoites present in the salivary glands of a female anopheline mosquito may be 500,000. We have to remember, however, that there are not 50 oocysts on the midgut of every infected mosquito and that all the oocysts may not succeed in producing so many sporozoites. It has been estimated, nevertheless, that the salivary glands of a single female mosquito may contain at least 200,000 sporozoites. When we reflect that each of these sporozoites is theoretically capable of starting in the liver and blood of man the prodigious multiplication of the numbers of the parasite described in chapter 11, we get an idea of the efficiency of multiplication of the numbers of individuals produced by these parasites as a means of ensuring their survival in the world.

THE EFFECTS OF THE MALARIAL PARASITES ON MAN

The disease caused by the human malarial parasites is still one of the most serious of the diseases with which man is afflicted. The name given to it, malaria, is a combination of the Italian words *malo*, which means bad, and *aria*, which means air. It refers to the belief formerly held that the disease came from the bad air of the marshes and swamps in which, as we now know,

The Malarial Parasites

the mosquitoes which transmit the disease to man breed and multiply. The disease affected man in the earliest years of his history in Babylonia, Assyria, India, and South China, and it was well known in ancient Greece and Rome. In Rome and the Roman Campagna it became so prevalent that a Goddess of the tertian and quartan malarial fevers, the DEA FEBRIS, was worshipped in the hope of preventing and curing the disease. Some experts believe that the decline of the Greek and Roman civilizations was hastened by malaria, but others doubt this. During the Middle Ages malaria was prevalent in Europe and Asia and probably also in Africa, and it spread, during this period, to America, to which country it may have been taken by men who sailed to America with Columbus in 1493. Between 1661 and 1664 there were severe epidemics of malaria in England. The disastrous effects of malaria, when it gets out of hand, have been many times exemplified by the epidemics of it that have, from time to time, occurred in various countries. They are well exemplified by the epidemics that occurred in Brazil between the years 1931 and 1938. A brief description of the disaster that then struck this country will show us how the disease may spread and how terrible its effects may be.

The seeds of this disastrous and comparatively recent calamity were sown when, late in 1929 and early in 1930, the mosquito, *Anopheles gambiae*, which is one of the chief vectors of malaria in tropical Africa, was transported, either by fast French destroyers travelling from the West African port of Dakar to Natal in Brazil, or by aeroplanes making the same journey, to the coast of Brazil at Natal. These mosquitoes, finding on the coast water in which they could breed, established themselves, first on the Brazilian coast and later in the interior of that country and they began to transmit malarial parasites already present in the blood of Brazilian people. The result was that there were epidemics of malaria in the city of Natal and efforts to control the mosquito were made. These efforts, however, began too late. The mosquito had begun to spread slowly into the country and its spread continued throughout the years 1932 to 1937. By 1938 it was being transported by vehicles travelling northwards and perhaps also

by boats plying along the coast, to the States of Rio Grande do
Norte and Ceará, in which the mosquitoes found, not only
favourable conditions for their breeding, but also a population
who were ill-nourished and were therefore not fully resistant to
malaria.

There followed an epidemic of malaria that was as severe as
any known to history. In June 1938 some 200,000 people in
the State of Rio Grande do Norte were suffering from the disease and, later that year, the disease spread to the country
watered by the River Jaquaribe. The people here were
weakened by malnutrition, they had no money to buy remedies, and the death-rate was very high. Shortage of food and
incessant rains made the situation worse. By June 1938 practically the whole population was infected. Economic life was
disrupted. People who could leave the district did so, but they
took the parasites with them and so spread the disease to the
districts into which they fled. It was estimated that, between
April and October of the year 1938, about 100,000 people had
been infected and that 20,000 died. Nearly everyone in the
area was in mourning for lost relatives.

This is, of course, no worse a tale than many that can be
told of malaria. The story of the conquest of *Anopheles gambiae*, in Brazil, which was so complete that, by 1941, no speci-
men of *Anopheles gambiae* born in Brazil could be found during
that year, is one of the greatest of the many stories about the
conquest of disease. The details of this astonishing feat of control were recorded by Soper and Wilson (1943). A similar
feat was performed in Egypt a few years later when the same
mosquito invaded that country.

Malaria, happily, does not always cause disasters as severe
as the one that has just been briefly described. Its effects vary
according to the species of the parasite that causes them, and,
although the parasites may kill, *Plasmodium falciparum* being
especially dangerous, the general effect of the disease is, not
to kill large numbers of people, but either to weaken the resistance of people to other diseases, or to stunt, as the hookworms also do, their mental and physical development and to
shorten the duration of their lives. The disease may, however,

be the cause of the deaths of many children. Its economic and social effects and its effects on agriculture and industry may be severe. As Sinton (1935) wrote: 'The problem of existence in very many parts of India is the problem of malaria. There is no aspect of life in the country which is not affected, either directly or indirectly, by this disease. It constitutes one of the most important causes of economic misfortune, engendering poverty, diminishing the quantity and quality of the food supply, lowering the physical and intellectual standard of the nation, and hampering increased prosperity and economic progress in every way.'

Some actual estimates of the financial cost of the disease are given by the *Chronicle of the World Health Organization* (1955). Howard (1909) estimated that, in 1908, malaria was costing the U.S.A. 100 million dollars a year and Williams (1938) estimated that in 1938 the annual cost had risen to 500 million dollars. Even now, says W.H.O., when malaria is rare in the U.S.A., it still imposes an enormous hidden tax on that country, because imports of goods, such as 'basic minerals, hardwoods, coffee, cocoa and vegetable oils' which come from malarious areas, cost the U.S.A. 5 per cent more than they would if the cost of malaria control in the exporting countries were not necessary. Alternatively, lack of malaria control may be an even greater expense to these countries; and American markets in these countries may be smaller because of the financial burden of malaria control.

Balfour and Scott (1924) calculated that the direct annual cost of sickness and death due to malaria in India was between 50 and 60 million pounds sterling. These figures do not include the indirect losses inflicted by the disease.

More recently, in southern Egypt in 1942–3, an epidemic of malaria cost one plantation alone the equivalent of 600,000 American dollars; half the wheat and a third of the sugar-cane crops were lost, because most of the labourers were too ill with chills and fever to harvest them.

For governments malaria poses many serious problems. It faces them with diminished reserves from taxation, increased costs for medical care, demands for higher wages in dangerous areas, slower development of natural resources, retarded social development, and less efficient leadership. The problems presented by malaria to commanders of armies in the field are so serious that the first priority has to be given to them. In the Second World War malaria was a top-priority problem in the Mediterranean, India, Burma, and the South Pacific areas. As Chandler (1955) points out, it caused, in the South Pacific campaign, five times as many casualties as the actual fighting did. It was necessary to beat the mosquitoes before the Japanese could be taken on. Fairley (1947) estimated that the casualties caused by malaria in the south-west Pacific area between September 1943 and February 1944 amounted to about 60·8 per cent of the forces in action in that area. In earlier wars malaria has been a no less serious enemy. In 1916, for instance, about a quarter of the British Macedonian force of some 123,000 men had to be taken into hospital and treated for malaria and the French troops suffered similar effects. Their enemies, the Germans, also suffered to much the same degree, so that fighting became impossible. Further information about the effects of malaria upon various wars in history is given by Lapage (1950), who also discusses in this article the effects upon war of various other parasites.

Malaria begins, as probably everyone knows, with a chill, accompanied by shivering and other symptoms, and this is quickly followed by fever, which ends with profuse sweating. These symptoms constitute what is called an 'attack' of malaria, and the attacks follow one another at the intervals of time explained below until the infected person becomes free of symptoms. The attacks of malaria do not begin until the multiplication of the parasites in the blood has produced a certain concentration of them there. They are caused by the bursting of the red cells of the blood and the liberation, not only of the merozoites, but of the products of the destruction of the red blood cells. Probably these sensitize the infected person, so that the chill, fever and other symptoms are allergic reactions on his part. Because the attacks of malaria are caused by the liberation of these substances into the blood, they coincide with the multiple divisions of the parasites and this is the reason

168

why the terms 'tertian' and 'quartan' are used to describe the forms of malaria caused by the different species of the parasites. As Chandler (1955) explains, they are based on the Roman practice of counting the day on which something happens as the first of a series of days. The multiple divisions of *Plasmodium vivax* typically occur every forty-eight hours, so that, by this Roman method of calculating the days, attacks of malaria caused by this species occur typically every third day and the malaria caused by *P. vivax* is therefore called *tertian* malaria. The schizogony of *Plasmodium malariae*, on the other hand, occurs about every seventy-two hours, so that the attacks of malaria caused by this species occur about every fourth day and the malaria is said to be quartan in consequence. The schizogony of *Plasmodium falciparum* is less regular, but it is predominantly tertian. Because the effects of this species are more severe than those of the other species, and may be fatal, the disease it causes is sometimes called malignant tertian malaria, or subtertian or pernicious malaria, in contrast to the disease caused by *P. vivax*, which is called benign tertian malaria. The disease caused by *P. falciparum* is also called aestivo-autumnal fever, because infections occur in the summer and autumn.

The explanation just given of the terms tertian and quartan is adequate to describe what happens in simple uncomplicated infections with single species of the malarial parasites and in people who have never suffered from the disease before. It is not, however, adequate to explain what happens in the majority of people. We have to remember that, although the multiple divisions of the four species of the malarial parasites typically occur at the intervals of time stated, so that the attacks of malaria are typically tertian or quartan, the infected person may suffer malarial attacks more frequently than this. One reason for this is that two successive infections may occur, so that there may be two broods of malarial parasites multiplying in the blood at the same time. Because their cycles of multiplication overlap, the attacks of malaria may occur, not every three days, but more often. People infected with *Plasmodium vivax*, may, for this reason, have malarial attacks every

169

day, so that their malaria is *quotidian*, not tertian. This may go on for several days, but, later in the course of the disease, the cycles of multiplication of the two broods of parasites tend to occur at the same time, so that the malarial attacks become typically tertian. After attacks due to this primary infection have gone on for two weeks to a month, the attacks abate, but there may be relapses for as long as three years.

Daily (quotidian) attacks of malaria are especially likely to occur in people infected with *Plasmodium falciparum*. This species is more likely than the other species to depart from the tertian periodicity of its multiple division in the blood, partly because the periodicity of its cycles of multiplication in the blood is less regular than that of the other species and partly because more than two broods of the parasites may be present. The result is that attacks of malaria may occur either every day, or, if more than two broods of parasites are present, twice in one day. The fever caused by this species, is therefore often irregular and it may be continuous; it may go on for a fortnight or so and there may be relapses of it for two to nine months after that. The periodicity of the fever may be further altered by the fact that infection with *Plasmodium vivax* may be present as well as infection with *P. falciparum*.

Infections with *Plasmodium malariae* may also at first cause daily attacks of fever, but the attacks are milder than those caused by the other species. They become typically quartan and last for a month or two; but this species is especially likely to cause relapses and these may go on for several years; it is known that they may go on, in some people, for twenty years.

Infections with *Plasmodium ovale* are the mildest of all. Attacks of malaria caused by it are usually tertian and they may last only a few days. The infection may then end without subsequent relapses. Because the attacks of malaria are tertian, infections with this species may be mistaken for infections with *Plasmodium vivax*.

The onset of the fever in persons infected with *P. vivax*, *P. malariae*, and *P. ovale* is usually sudden and it begins with the well-known chill and fever which goes on for several hours and then ends with profuse sweating. In persons infected with

170

P. falciparum the initial chill is not so marked and the fever is more prolonged. Infections with this species are more dangerous and may be fatal. The infected person may be unconscious and cold, or comatose and restless, and the parasites may get into the blood vessels of the brain, producing a cerebral type of the disease; they may then cause the red blood cells to clump together, so that a small blood vessel of the brain may be blocked by them and symptoms like these of a 'stroke' may occur; in other types of infections with this species there may be bleeding from the skin or the mucous membranes, or there may be severe vomiting, diarrhoea, or symptoms like those of acute dysentery.

Attacks of malaria are, whatever the species that causes them, preceded by an *incubation period* during which the parasites are multiplying, first in the liver and later in the blood. This incubation period varies for several reasons. First it varies according to the species of malarial parasite concerned. The incubation period of malaria caused by *P. vivax* is 9 to 17 days (average 15 days) and that of malaria caused by *P. ovale* is similar. The incubation periods of malaria caused by *P. falciparum* is 8 to 14 days and that of malaria caused by *P. malariae* about 18 days. The duration of the incubation period varies, however, according to the size of the dose of sporozoites received and the immunity (resistance) to the parasites which people develop once they have been infected. Because this resistance may be reduced or broken down by poor nutrition or other diseases which affect the general health of the infected person, malnutrition and other diseases may also affect the incubation period of malaria.

The size of the dose of sporozoites is important because, as Hoare (1949) explains, when a mosquito's salivary glands are full of sporozoites, it will, when it first sucks human blood, inject into the first person bitten by it thousands of sporozoites, so that this person receives a big dose of them. The resistance of this person may then be relatively quickly overcome and the incubation period of the disease may be only seven days or so.

At subsequent feeds, however, the mosquito's salivary

glands contain fewer sporozoites, so that persons bitten then receive fewer individual malarial parasites. Their resistance may then be better able to deal with the parasites. They may, if their resistance is high, hold the parasites in check, so that they suffer only mild malaria, or even no symptoms at all. If their resistance is, in fact, overcome after all, this may take longer than usual, so that the incubation period is prolonged for several months.

When the disease is established, its subsequent course will depend on the species of the parasite that causes it, on the strain within that species that is involved, on the size of the initial dose of sporozoites received by the sufferer and on the resistance (immunity) that man develops to the disease and to further infections with it.

The way in which resistance acts may be better understood if we try to calculate what might happen if each of the sporozoites infected by the mosquito were allowed by the human body to develop without a check.

First it would multiply its numbers in the liver – and perhaps also in other organs as well. The thousands of merozoites thus produced would then be liberated into the blood. As Hoare (1949) explains, each of these merozoites, would, if it were a merozoite of *P. vivax*, give rise to 24 merozoites every 24 hours, and at this rate, it would produce in 14 days, 200 to 300 million malarial parasites. If this rate of multiplication went on without a check, the infected person could not live very long. Chandler (1955) quotes a similar calculation made by Knowles, who estimated that a single malarial parasite that produced 20 merozoites every time it underwent schizogony, would produce, in 20 days, so many parasites that there would be about 4 in every red blood cell in the human body, provided that the infected person lived as long as this. But all people infected with malarial parasites do not die within 20 days. What is it that prevents the parasites from multiplying in the manner described above? The answer to this question has been provided largely by the study of the malarial parasites of birds. It can be stated in the single word immunity.

The Malarial Parasites

When an uninfected person is infected with malarial parasites his body begins at once, or almost at once, to attack the invaders. The cells of the body that carry out the attack are the phagocytic cells. The entry of the malarial parasites into the body stimulates an enormous production of phagocytic cells, particularly of those that are produced in the liver, spleen, and bone marrow. These organs therefore become enlarged and this is one of the reasons why enlargement of the liver and spleen are characteristic of malaria. The phagocytes attack and engulf the red cells of the blood that contain the malarial parasites and they destroy both the parasites and the red blood cells. The destruction of red blood cells that occurs in malaria is thus due not only to destruction of them by the malarial parasites, but also to destruction of parasitized red cells by the sufferer's own phagocytes. It is not surprising, therefore, that anaemia is one of the features of chronic malaria.

The immunity developed by man against his malarial parasites is well exemplified by the natives of malarious countries, who have lived in these countries for generations and have been exposed to repeated infections with malarial parasites. Some of these natives have, in consequence, developed a high resistance to malaria and are troubled much less by it than white or other immigrants into these malarious areas are. American negroes, for instance, suffer only a mild disease when they are infected by *P. vivax*. The immunity developed against the malarial parasites is specific. It protects, that is to say, only against the species of malarial parasite that causes man to develop it. Infection with *P. vivax* causes the development only of immunity to this species and this immunity does not protect man against *P. falciparum*, *P. malariae*, or *P. ovale*. Immunity to these species develops only when infections with them occur.

Immunity to malaria is, obviously, never natural; if it were, man would never suffer from malaria. It is, therefore, always acquired, and is influenced, like the immunity developed by man and other animals to some other kinds of parasitic animals, by a number of factors that operate on the host of the

173

parasitic animal. We have seen that it is more effective in certain races of people who have been for long exposed to malaria. It is also influenced by the age of the infected person, young people and children usually showing less resistance than older people do, so that they suffer more. This is an example of the general rule that young hosts suffer more than older ones. Resistance to malaria is also reduced, as resistance to most diseases is, by factors that reduce the general state of the health of the host. The brief account given above of the disastrous effects of malaria in northern Brazil is a good example of the general rule that the resistance to malaria of under-nourished or otherwise badly-fed peoples is much reduced.

MODES OF INFECTION WITH MALARIA

Although man is usually infected with malaria by the bites of mosquitoes, other modes of infection are possible. Rarely, for instance, unborn children may be infected with malarial parasites that are in the mother's blood. Usually the placenta in the womb, through which the unborn child gets its nourishment from the mother, effectively keeps the parasites out of the child's blood, but instances are known in which this barrier fails. Probably this happens only when the placenta has been damaged by disease or in some other way. There are also instances of children being infected by mosquitoes that bite them immediately after they have been born, or even while they are being born. Infection acquired in this way is easily confused with the relatively few instances that are known of infection of the child from the maternal blood before it is ready to be born.

Another way in which infection may be acquired is through blood transfusions. These may occur when the blood has been stored for as long as two weeks. People addicted to giving themselves drugs, such as heroin, by hypodermic syringes, often infect each other by using insufficiently sterilized syringes immediately after these have been used by a person infected with malarial parasites.

The Malarial Parasites

The Geographical Distribution of Malaria

Malaria, whatever form it takes, is a cosmopolitan disease. Its geographical distribution is, of course, determined by the habits and geographical distribution of the various species of anopheline mosquitoes in whose bodies the sexual phases of the life histories of the malarial parasites must occur, but one or more species of these mosquitoes are able to breed in most parts of the world. They cannot breed at altitudes above 9,000 feet and for this reason malaria is absent from those altitudes. In parts of the world in which the anopheline mosquito is not able to live and breed, malaria cannot occur. For this reason the disease is, in fact, less common in mountainous regions and also in deserts, in which lack of water inhibits the breeding of the mosquitoes. It is also absent from New Zealand, Hawaii, Fiji, the Gilbert and Ellice Islands, Samoa, and the Marquesas and it is not found north of latitude 60° N. or south of latitude 30° S. These areas free from malaria represent, however, a relatively small part of the world and the disease is found pretty well everywhere else, though its prevalence in particular areas is variable. It is common in coastal areas and in some parts of the world it is *hyperendemic*, a term which means that its incidence is much higher than it is in *endemic* areas in which it is always present. The chief areas in which it is hyperendemic are Southern China, Indo-China and Malaya, the East Indies, India, Asia Minor and Southern Russia, Central and South America, the West Indies, the Solomon Islands, the New Hebrides, and the northern coast of Australia.

The incidence of the four species of the malarial parasites also varies. *Plasmodium vivax* is the most widely distributed species and it prevails in the temperate zones of the world, probably because it can develop in the mosquito at lower climatic temperatures than the other species are able to. This species is indigenous, that is to say, it can be acquired by healthy persons from mosquitoes infected in the indigenous

175

area, as far north in Europe as Southern Sweden and Lake Ladoga in Russia and as far south as southern Queensland, South Africa, and northern Argentina. It was reported in 1946 from northern Ireland, where a healthy person was infected by mosquitoes that had become infected in that country. *P. falciparum* occurs especially in subtropical and tropical zones and is rarer in temperate zones. It is present in most tropical countries and in Southern Europe. *P. malariae* is widespread, but its distribution is more localized than that of the other species. It is found in the Mediterranean countries, Syria, Iraq, Palestine, India, Malaya, Central and Southern China, the Philippine Islands, New Guinea, the West Indies, Brazil, Panama and Central America, the Southern United States, and Central and West Africa. The exact distribution of *P. ovale* is not known, but it occurs in East and West Africa, Rhodesia and the Belgian Congo, in Russia, China and Central Asia, the Philippine Islands, Persia, India, Central America, and the west coast of South America.

The habits of the females of the species of the genus *Anopheles* have much influence on the spread of malaria. It is known that the human malarial parasites can undergo their sexual cycle (sporogony) in over 100 species of this genus; but the number of species that are really important vectors of the disease is more of the order of twenty or thirty; and some species or strains of malarial parasites develop better in some species of mosquitoes than in others. It will, therefore, be readily understood that different species of mosquitoes are important in different areas. In Egypt, Arabia, and tropical Africa, for instance, *Anopheles gambiae* is the chief vector of the disease, though in tropical Africa *A. funestus* is also important. In Polynesia and the Australian region *A. punctulatus* is the chief mosquito involved. In Central America and down to the Argentine it is *A. darlingi*. In Holland, Spain, and Portugal the chief vector is *A. maculipennis atroparvus*; in Southern Europe, *A. superpictus*; and in India, *A. stephensi*, *A. sundaicus*, and *A. minimus* are involved.

The species of mosquitoes have different breeding and other habits and vary in their capacities of feeding on human blood. Some, for instance, breed in brackish rather than fresh water and this limits their geographical distribution. There are, moreover, races within certain species whose habits differ. Thus the European species *A. maculipennis* includes several races that only rarely suck human blood, so that they are not important vectors of human malaria. Other races of this species, on the other hand, do feed upon man and are important vectors of the disease. Malaria-carrying mosquitoes also vary in their other relations with man, some entering human dwellings readily, while others attack man more often outside. Species that enter buildings to rest after feeding are more readily reached by DDT or other sprays directed against them, so this kind of habit is important from the point of view of control.

All these factors – the number of sporozoites received through the mosquito bite, the age, health, race, and resistance of the person bitten, the species or strain of the parasite and of the mosquito, and the habits of the mosquitoes themselves – influence the incidence of malaria in different parts of the world. The establishment and persistence of the disease in particular areas may be determined, even in areas in which the right mosquito-hosts are present, by the average number of bites per person inflicted on the people living in those areas. Quite slight changes in this average number of bites per person may cause the decline of the disease or even its disappearance from the area. Chandler (1955) suggests that this has happened recently in the United States, where the numbers of mosquitoes that transmit malaria have been reduced by spraying with insecticides and by other measures taken against them to such an extent that the number of feeds of human blood necessary to maintain the parasites became no longer possible, with the result that malaria has been virtually eradicated from the United States.

The difficulties that confront the malarial parasites are indeed many and a brief enumeration of them here will help us to understand what conditions must be fulfilled before the disease caused by these parasites can spread. The mosquitoes, of course, need water in which their larvae must develop. They also need, when they are adult insects, a certain degree of humidity and without this they cannot live. If they are to spread malaria, the female mosquito must take up, when she sucks human blood, both male and female gametocytes of the parasites and she must take up enough of these to establish an infection in her body. This she cannot always do, because there may not be many gametocytes in the blood of man at certain times and enough of them may not be present in persons who have developed an immunity to the disease. Once the infection has been established in a mosquito, a certain number of days must pass before sporozoites are produced and during this period the mosquito cannot transmit malaria. There are, moreover, biological races within the various species of mos-

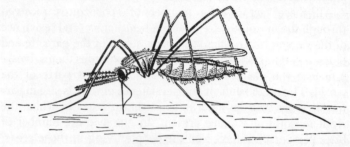

Fig. 41. A female mosquito sucking blood

quitoes and some of these are more readily infected with some species of the malarial parasites, or with some strains within those species, than with others. Thus English workers found that *Anopheles maculipennis* in England can be infected with a strain of *P. falciparum* obtained from Italy, but not with a strain obtained from India. Some races of mosquitoes can, moreover, establish infections with some species or strains of malarial parasites by a single blood-sucking act, whereas several acts of blood-sucking are required to establish infections with other strains or species of the parasites. Another factor which restricts the power of the female mosquito to transmit malaria is the fact, already mentioned above, that the sexual cycle of the parasites in the mosquito can be completed only when the temperature of the environment of the mosquito remains within certain maximum and minimum limits and these limits vary with the different species of the parasites. These limits of the external temperature have been given above and in some climates the necessary environmental temperature is not maintained for the time required for the completion of the sexual cycle in the mosquito. In the parts of England, for instance, in which malaria used to be prevalent – in, that is to say, East Anglia and along the coast as far as the Isle of Wight, and in certain other, more isolated areas – one of the factors that prevent the outbreak of serious epidemics of malaria is the fact that the climatic temperature, even in the summer, is only rarely high enough or long enough to allow the sexual cycle of the malarial parasites to be completed. There are plenty of mosquitoes capable of transmitting the parasites and there are – at any rate at certain times – people in England with malarial parasites in their blood; but the mosquitoes are, so to speak, kept too cold and sporozoites cannot develop in them. Nevertheless it may happen occasionally that they do develop in English mosquitoes and that English people are then infected by malarial parasites taken up by the mosquitoes from the blood of English people. This happened, for instance, after the First World War, when many soldiers came back to England with malarial parasites in their blood; and there is always the risk that the right conditions may occur for it to happen again. The fact that an indigenous case of malaria occurred in Northern Ireland in 1946 has been mentioned above. The species that English people are most likely to acquire is *P. vivax*, because the sexual cycle of this species can be completed in the mosquito at lower temperatures than the sexual cycles of the other species of the parasites can. This interesting question of the factors which govern the occurrence of malaria in England has been discussed by McNalty (1943), Lapage (1951), and others. It is linked with the factors which govern the greater prevalence of malaria in countries as near to England as Holland and other northern European countries, and the study of the incidence of the disease in these comparatively northerly countries teaches us a great deal about the factors which govern the geographical distribution of the disease.

THE CONTROL OF MALARIA

In a book of this size only a brief outline of the complex problem of malaria control can be given. For detailed accounts of it the reader is referred to Chandler (1955), Craig and Faust (1955), Boyd (1949), and the books and papers mentioned by these authors. For a brief account of the importance of malaria, its geographical distribution at the present time and of recent successes in banishing it from some parts of the world, the reader is referred to the *Chronicle of the World Health Organization* (1955).

The methods used to control malaria may be divided into those which are directed against the mosquitoes which transmit the parasites to man and those which are directed against the parasites when they are in the human body.

One of the earliest methods used against the mosquitoes was drainage of the areas in which the disease was prevalent. The object of this method is to prevent, or at any rate to handicap, the breeding of the mosquitoes. Drainage was used in ancient Rome and various Caesars tried to drain the Pontine marshes, but this was not successfully done until 1940, when reclamation of land created, in place of an area in which, in 1930, not a single permanent human household could be found, 200,000 acres of farmland, on which 50,000 people were able to support themselves. From the twentieth century onwards antimalarial drainage has been a feature of measures taken against the disease in many parts of the world. Drainage is, however, expensive and it does not guarantee full control. The mosquitoes have, as other animals have, a way of avoiding the measures taken against them. They still find breeding places in the small ditches and canals that remain. Measures of this kind have, therefore, to be supplemented by other measures.

Among these additional measures are attacks on the larvae of the mosquitoes with such substances as Paris Green, which kills the larvae, or with petroleum oils spread over water-surfaces, which prevent the larvae from getting the air that they must have. Methods of this kind were used, for instance, on a large scale in the campaign against *Anopheles gambiae* in Brazil mentioned above. They can, as that campaign showed, be very effective, but they are expensive and laborious. They are more suitable for small areas. Nowadays the method more often used is to attack the adult mosquitoes rather than the larvae.

The adult mosquitoes are killed with insecticides sprayed on to the interior of houses and other buildings used by man and also all over every part of aeroplanes and other means of human transport. It is, in fact, nowadays standard practice thus to spray long-range aeroplanes and also to search them meticulously for mosquitoes that may be resting in them. Among the insecticides used DDT has been, until recently, the most effective. Its action persists on the surfaces on to which it is sprayed, so that mosquitoes which escape the direct spray may be killed by it later on. Unfortunately mosquitoes, like house flies and some other species of two-winged flies, become resistant to DDT. Strains of them appear which are not killed by it and these strains continue to transmit the malarial parasites. Similar resistant strains of the mosquitoes which transmit yellow fever to man have also appeared and the fleas which transmit plague and the human body-lice which transmit typhus fever to man are also becoming resistant. DDT is not, for this reason, nowadays so reliable as it used to be and it may happen that we shall not, in the future, be able to use it as effectively as we have done in the past. Benzene hexachloride (BHC), Dieldrin, Chlordane, and other substances are, however, already being used effectively against ticks and other blood-sucking arthropods that have become resistant to DDT, and there is little doubt that biochemical research will provide us with additional effective insecticides and acaricides which will increase our control of all the arthropod vectors of disease.

The other chief method of controlling malaria is the use of drugs which will kill the parasites while they are in the body of man. The first of these antimalarial drugs to be used effectively was quinine. It is said that its efficacy was discovered

Animals Parasitic in Man

when, in 1638, the Countess d'El Cinchón, wife of the Viceroy of Peru, was cured of malaria by taking a preparation made from the barks of trees that contained quinine, and quinine was for this reason named Cinchóna. Thereafter quinine was our chief means of treating the disease. It is still a valuable antimalarial drug and is preferred by some experts for the treatment of severe infections with *Plasmodium falciparum*. Laboratory workers, however, have, in recent years, discovered other antimalarial drugs and the search for these was stimulated by the capture by the Japanese during the Second World War of the world's chief supplies of quinine.

We now have, as the result of the research that is always going on, a number of antimalarial drugs which can be made in the laboratory. They all have specific uses and limitations and their use must be controlled by experts experienced in the treatment of infections with the different especies of malarial parasites. Their various advantages and disadvantages, and the risks associated with their use, cannot be considered here. They are discussed by Covell *et al.* (1955).

Measures taken for the control of malaria include, in addition to control of the mosquitoes and treatment of infected people with antimalarial drugs, efforts to improve the nutrition and general health of populations in malarious areas. These are necessary because malnutrition and poor health arising from any cause not only reduce the capacity of the people to develop the immunity to malaria, but also undermine immunity that has already been developed. Good nutrition and good general health are therefore important means of supporting man's natural defences against the disease.

The results of energetic application of the methods of control just outlined have been, in recent years, remarkable. Beginning, as our battle with this calamitous disease did, with the discovery, by Laveran in 1880, of the parasites themselves, it was greatly advanced when Ross, in 1898, discovered that the malarial parasites of birds were transmitted by mosquitoes, and when Grassi and his colleagues independently worked out, and published later in the same year, the life history of the human malarial parasites in the bodies of female mosquitoes of

182

the genus *Anopheles*. The discovery of DDT and the newer in-secticides that will kill the mosquitoes further advanced our control over malaria and nowadays the disease has been entirely, or almost entirely, banished from some parts of the world. Thus it has been eliminated from the United States, Italy, Sicily, Sardinia, Corsica, Crete, and Cyprus and it is being vigorously combated in Brazil, British and French Guiana, Greece, Israel, Yugoslavia, Venezuela, Madagascar, and north-eastern Australia. It is nowadays absent from much of Argentina and Chile. Chile, which was the first country to eradicate it, did so before DDT and its action on the adult mosquitoes were known, by attacking the larvae, as was done during the outbreak in Brazil described above. In large areas of Bombay, Mysore, and Ceylon, modern control has almost completely prevented the infection of man. In most other afflicted countries energetic campaigns against it, most of them assisted by the World Health Organization, are in progress. Constant vigilance is, however, needed to make sure that the disease does not return to areas from which it has been eradicated.

There is, moreover, much still to be done. The World Health Organization (1955) reports that intense malaria is still found in parts of the Americas between latitudes 15° N. and 15° S. and in Asia south of 40° N. and also in Indonesia, Africa, and the south-west Pacific region. The map published by this authority (1955) gives a graphic picture of the progress of our conquest of the disease, but it is, nevertheless, clear that malaria still causes more illness and economic loss than any other human malady does. To quote the World Health Organization (1955) again, more than 250 million of the 2,500 million or so people in the world, that is to say, about 1 in 10, have a clinical attack of malaria every year and possibly $2\frac{1}{2}$ million people die of malaria every year. So long as this is true, we can hardly abate our war on these parasites, which have, in spite of all the natural difficulties with which they have to contend, maintained themselves so successfully and have so effectively defeated all the measures that man has been able to take against them.

CHAPTER NINE

The Human Trypanosomes

TH E human trypanosomes, like the human malarial parasites, are single-celled Protozoa; but they live, not inside the red blood cells, as the malarial parasites do, but in the fluid part (*plasma*) of the blood. They are therefore extracellular, not intracellular, parasites. They belong to the group of Protozoa called the Flagellata (Mastigophora), all of which move by means of a whip-like extension of the body-protoplasm called a flagellum. As figs. 42A and 43 show, a trypanosome has an elongated, rather flattened and somewhat spindle-shaped body, inside which there is, as there is in every typical cell, a nucleus that governs the life of the cell. The nucleus of a trypanosome is called the *trophonucleus*, which means that it is concerned with the nutrition and general life of the cell. In addition to this nucleus, however, there is another structure, called the *kinetoplast* (*kinetonucleus*) which looks rather like a second nucleus, but is, in fact, a structure concerned with the management, so to speak, of the single flagellum, which is the locomotor organ of the trypanosome. This kinetoplast is always near the *posterior* end of the trypanosome, or, at any rate, nearer that end than the anterior end. The flagellum arises near to it and there is, at or near its point of origin, a small granule, called the *basal granule*. From this the flagellum passes *forwards* along the body of the trypanosome to become, as a rule, free beyond the anterior end. Along its length the flagellum is bound to the trypanosome's body by a flange, or ribbon, of protoplasm called the *undulating membrane*. When the trypanosome is moving about in the fluid part of the blood, the flagellum and its undulating membrane perform wave-like movements which move the trypanosome along. This loco-motor apparatus of the trypanosome has possibly evolved in response to the need to move about in a relatively viscid fluid like the blood.

Trypanosomes are descended, without any doubt, from non-parasitic flagellate Protozoa which have only one flagellum arising at the anterior end (fig. 42) and a single nucleus. From these the first step was to the species belonging to the genus *Crithidia,* shown in fig. 42B, which are parasitic in the food canals of the daddy-long-legs and other insects. In these

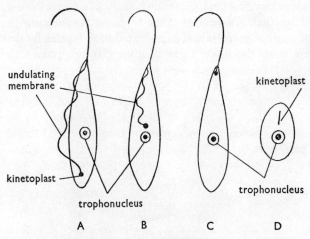

undulating membrane

kinetoplast

kinetoplast

trophonucleus

trophonucleus

A   B   C   D

Fig. 42. Diagrams of (A) *Trypanosoma,* (B) *Crithidia,*
(C) *Leptomonas,* (D) *Leishmania*

species the origin of the flagellum has moved backwards down the body, a short undulating membrane connecting it with the body has developed and the flagellum is governed by a kine-toplast, which is, however, still in front of the trophonucleus. If we imagine that the origin of the flagellum has moved still further back, so that it lies in the posterior region of the body, and that, for this reason, the undulating membrane extends along the whole length of the body, we arrive at the structure of the trypanosome.

How do we know that this is not merely a speculation about the origin of the trypanosomes? We know because we know that every animal tends to show, in the course of its life history, some of the features of its ancestors. The frog, for example, which belongs to the group of vertebrates called the Amphibia, lives, while it is a tadpole, like the fish from which the Amphibia were derived; and even man, for a brief part of his life in the womb, has, in his neck, gill-slits, like those of a fish. Occasionally, in fact, these gill-slits fail to close and the child is born with them in its neck. If, knowing this fact that animals recapitulate in the development of the individual their ancestral history, we look at the life history of a trypanosome, what do we find? We find that the trypanosome, during the phase of its development in the food canal of the tsetse fly that transmits it to the blood of man, goes through phases the

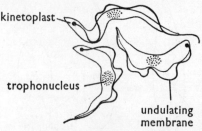

kinetoplast

trophonucleus

undulating
membrane

Fig. 43. *Trypanosoma gambiense. Trypanosoma rhodesiense* is similar

structure of which is like that of the species of the genus *Crithidia* described above. Some species of trypanosomes also show, during their development, a small, pear-shaped phase (fig. 42D) without a flagellum at all; and, because it has no flagellum, it has no undulating membrane either. The kinetoplast however, remains and of course the trophonucleus, because without this the cell could not live. These phases are called *leishmanial phases*, because their structure is like that of the human parasites belonging to the genus *Leishmania* (fig. 47) described below, which cause, in the tropics, the disease called kala-azar and also the ulcers on the skin called tropical sores, or Baghdad boils. These species are named after Sir W. Leishman who discovered them. During their life histories they also show crithidial phases, so that these genera, and others that are parasitic in insects and in the latex of some plants, but not in man, all belong to a group of species closely related to each other.

Three species of the genus *Trypanosoma* cause the disease of man which will, in this book, be called trypanosomiasis. This name is better because the colloquial name, sleeping sickness, can be applied to other diseases as well and, in any event, somnolence is not always a feature of the disease caused by trypanosomes. The three species of trypanosomes that cause human trypanosomiasis are: *Trypanosoma gambiense* and *T. rhodesiense* (fig. 43), which cause trypanosomiasis of man in Africa only, where they are transmitted to man chiefly by tsetse flies (fig. 44), which exist only in Africa; and *Trypanosoma cruzi*, which differs in important respects from the other two species and causes a different disease of man in South America, especially in Brazil, where it is transmitted to man by blood-sucking bugs, related to, but very different from, the bed-bug.

Let us consider the African species first.

Trypanosoma gambiense

This species has possibly been derived from *T. brucei*, which causes trypanosomiasis of horses, camels, pigs, and monkeys (except the baboon) and a milder form of the disease in cattle, sheep, and goats. *T. gambiense* infects man in tropical West Africa and areas near Lake Tchad, in the Southern Sudan, on Lake Victoria, and also in French Equatorial Africa and the Belgian Congo. It is inoculated into man chiefly by tsetse flies, in the food canals of which it must undergo a series of changes before these flies can transmit it back to man. The tsetse flies are two-winged flies (Diptera) related to the stable flies and house flies rather than to the horse flies. Both male and female tsetse flies suck blood, so that both sexes can transmit the trypanosomes. In this respect the tsetse flies differ from the mosquitoes which transmit malaria. All the tsetse flies belong to the genus *Glossina* and several species of these flies can transmit *T. gambiense* to man. The species most important as vectors of *T. gambiense* are *Glossina palpalis*, *G. pallidipes*, and, in northern Nigeria *G. tachinoides*. Other species of the genus *Glossina* may, however, act as vectors. These tsetse flies pick up *T. gambiense* chiefly from other human beings, but it may lie up in wild pig in West Africa and in the sheep, goat, and cattle, so that these animals may be reservoir hosts, from which the infection can be derived.

Trypanosoma rhodesiense

This species, the structure of which is not essentially different from that of *T. gambiense*, is probably a strain of *T. brucei*

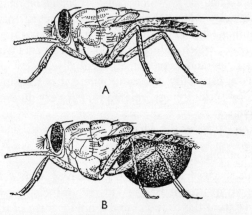

Fig. 44. A tsetse fly (*Glossina* sp.). (A) unfed; (B) full of blood

which has become adapted to life in human blood. It attacks man in East and South-East Africa from Southern Rhodesia and Eastern Mozambique up to Uganda and inland to Tanganyika and the Eastern Congo. Typically it causes in man a disease that follows a more rapid course and is more likely to be fatal than the disease caused by *T. gambiense*. This species occurs also in wild African hoofed animals (Ungulata), from which tsetse flies may transmit it to man.

Like *T. gambiense*, it is transmitted to man chiefly by tsetse flies (fig. 44). The species most concerned on the transmission of *T. rhodesiense* are *Glossina morsitans*, *G. pallidipes*, and, in certain areas, such as Tanganyika, *G. swynnertoni*; but other species may be vectors of it.

The Human Trypanosomes

Both *Trypanosoma gambiense* and *T. rhodesiense* multiply their numbers, in the plasma of human blood, by longitudinal division of their bodies. Most species of trypanosomes do this in the blood of their vertebrate hosts, though they do not all do it continuously, as *T. gambiense* and *T. rhodesiense* do. This process of division begins with division of the basal granule of the flagellum and the kinetoplast. One of the two products of the division keeps the old flagellum; in the other product of the division a new flagellum grows out of the half of the basal granule in it and a new undulating membrane is formed. Meanwhile the trophonucleus has divided into two, so that the organism now contains two sets of organs. The body then splits into two along its length, division beginning at the anterior end where the free part of the flagellum is. It is characteristic of these two species of trypanosomes and of some others, such as *T. evansi* and its relatives, *T. equinum* and *T. equiperdum*, that division of the trypanosomes in this manner produces in the blood of the vertebrate host trypanosomes that are either slender forms about 29 micra long with a tapering posterior end and a free flagellum at the other end, or short, stumpy forms, about 12 micra long, which usually have no free part of the flagellum at the anterior end; or forms intermediate between these about 23 micra long with a free flagellum. It is these forms which are taken up by the tsetse fly when it sucks human blood.

Usually, when *T. gambiense* and *T. rhodesiense* are sucked up by a tsetse fly, they undergo, in the food canal and salivary glands of the fly, a cycle of changes, which includes a further multiplication of their numbers by longitudinal division. The details of the changes that occur during their cycle need not be given here. Briefly it can be said that the first change is that a trypanosome appears in which the undulating membrane is not so pronounced and the kinetoplast is further forward, though still behind the trophonucleus. These forms multiply their numbers in the insect's food canal for about ten days, so that enormous numbers of them may be produced. Then more slender forms of them appear and these collect in the region of the tsetse fly's proventriculus, which is a pear-shaped dilatation of the anterior end of the middle part of the insect's food

189

canal. From this situation they move forward to the insect's gullet and from this reach the proboscis. From the proboscis they turn back again up the duct of the salivary gland, which discharges the saliva on a part of the proboscis called the hypopharynx or tongue (see fig. 51). In this manner the trypanosomes reach the salivary glands. In these glands they attach themselves by means of their flagella to the cells of the salivary glands and there they become forms (fig. 42) the structure of which resembles that of the species of the genus *Crithidia* described above. In these forms, that is to say, the kinetoplast is in front of the trophonucleus and the undulating membrane is therefore short.

These *crithidial forms*, as they are called, multiply their numbers by longitudinal division and eventually the trypanosome structure, with the kinetonucleus at the posterior end of the body, is resumed. Because these later trypanosome forms are produced at the end of the cycle of changes in the insect, they are called *metacyclic* forms and they, and they alone, can again infect man. They are, therefore, the infective phases of the trypanosome. The whole cycle of changes inside the tsetse fly requires for its completion from 15 to 35 days. A tsetse fly that has taken up human blood containing trypanosomes cannot, for this reason, infect a new human host for 15 to 35 days. But probably a tsetse fly, once it has taken up trypanosomes, remains capable of transmitting them to man for the rest of its life, which lasts, on an average for about 3 weeks in dry weather and a few months in the wet season.

It does not follow, however, that, when tsetse flies take up blood containing trypanosomes, they always become infected with the trypanosomes. In many flies the trypanosomes die before they become the metacyclic forms that are alone capable of infecting man. It is probable, in fact, that the species of trypanosomes that infect man in Africa, namely *Trypanosoma gambiense* and *T. rhodesiense*, do not succeed in going through their cycle in more than ten per cent of the tsetse flies, and among wild flies caught the proportion of infected flies is usually not more than one per cent. The ability of the trypanosomes to develop in the tsetse flies is affected by various

factors. One of these is the temperature at which the tsetse flies
have developed, more flies being infected when this temperature has been high than when it has been low. The human being from whom the tsetse flies take up the infection also influences the success of the trypanosome in developing in the flies.
If, for instance, the flies take trypanosomes from a person suffering from the early stages of trypanosomiasis, the trypanosomes are more likely to complete their development in the

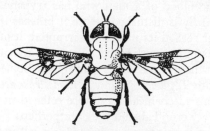

Fig. 45. A tabanid fly of the horse fly
type (*Tabanus* sp.)

flies than they are if they are taken up from a person who has
been suffering from chronic trypanosomiasis for some time.

The method of transmission of *T. gambiense* and *T. rhodesiense* just described is the usual one. Normally, that is to say,
the trypanosomes undergo, inside the flies, the cycle of
changes described and they cannot infect a new host until these
changes have been completed and the metacyclic forms of the
trypanosomes have been formed. This method of transmission
is, for this reason, called *cyclical transmission*. Both these species
of trypanosomes can, however, be transmitted by other methods. One of these methods is called *mechanical transmission*.
This term means that the trypanosomes are simply transferred
mechanically from the *blood* of one infected human being to the
blood of a healthy person by the proboscis of a blood-sucking
fly when it sucks the blood of man. When this happens, the
fly that transmits the trypanosomes need not be a tsetse fly.
Tabanid flies (fig. 45) of the horse fly type and the stable fly,
Stomoxys calcitrans, may, for instance, transmit trypanosomes
in this mechanical way. The proboscis of the fly acts, that is to

say, exactly as the needle of a hypodermic syringe, or any other instrument, would, if it were dipped into a culture of trypanosomes and then were thrust through the skin and entered the blood before it had had time to dry.

This is, in fact, what happens when *T. gambiense* or *T. rhodesiense* are transmitted mechanically. A cloud of tsetse flies may, for instance, follow a group of Negroes pulling off from the shore of an African river or lake in a canoe and one of them may suck the blood of a man who has trypanosomes in his blood. If that fly is disturbed before it finishes its meal, or if for any other reason its meal is interrupted, it may, while its proboscis is still wet with blood, bite one of the other Negroes and transmit the trypanosomes to his blood. Some experts consider that both *T. gambiense* and *T. rhodesiense* are transmitted to man in this mechanical way more often than we formerly thought they were. Tabanid flies are perhaps more likely to transmit them in this manner, because the cutting blades with which these flies puncture the skin inflict relatively coarse and irritating wounds, with the result that the person bitten reacts quickly and interrupts the fly's meal and drives it away, while its proboscis is still wet with blood, to finish its meal on the blood of somebody else.

Transmission by this mechanical method means, of course, that the cycle of changes and multiplication in the insect's food canal and salivary glands is omitted. One effect of this, if it were the normal method of infection of man, would be that the numbers of the trypanosomes available would be greatly reduced. This might not greatly affect the capacity of the trypanosomes to survive, because some species of trypanosomes that cause diseases of domesticated animals survive in spite of the fact that mechanical transmission is the only means by which they can pass from one host to another. *Trypanosoma evansi*, for example, which causes, in India, the disease of equines and dogs called surra and similar diseases of camels in Algeria and the Sudan, relies entirely on mechanical transmission by flies of the horse fly type (Tabanidae) and on the bites of the stable fly, *Stomoxys calcitrans*. Another species, *T. equinum*, which causes, in South America the disease called *mal de caderas* of horses, mules, sheep, goats, and cattle, also relies entirely on mechanical transmission by the same flies. It is the only species of trypanosome known which has no kinetoplast.

Although the human trypanosomes are usually transmitted to man by cyclical transmission through tsetse flies, and, less often, by mechanical transmission by tabanid flies and *Stomoxys*, it is known that *Trypanosoma gambiense* may be rarely transmitted from one human being to another by the sexual act and some experts believe that it can pass from an infected mother to her child either in the mother's milk or to the child while it is still in the mother's womb. It is not known whether *T. rhodesiense* may be transmitted in these unusual ways.

The disease caused by *T. gambiense* and *T. rhodesiense* cannot be described in any detail here. Typically *T. rhodesiense* causes a form of trypanosomiasis that has a more rapid course and may end, if it is not treated, within a year, in the death of the infected person. The disease caused by *T. gambiense* on the other hand, takes a slower course and may last several years. The disease is typically a disease of the lymphatic and nervous systems. At the site of the bite of the tsetse fly an elevated, hardened, and painful nodule appears and enlargement of the lymphatic glands in the neck and groin occurs. There is fever, with enlargement of the liver and spleen. There is, that is to say, a chronic inflammation of the lymphatic system and this inflammation spreads especially to the lymphatics of the brain and spinal cord. Until the fever begins, the infected person may not know that he has the disease; but then he suffers from headache, neuralgia, cramps, weakness in the legs, anaemia, shortness of breath, pain in the heart, and other symptoms. Later, when the inflammation spreads to the brain and spinal cord, the sufferer develops mental apathy, with excitable periods, muscle spasms, incoordination of movement, pain, and stiffness in the neck and sleepiness, which may be so pronounced that the patient falls asleep at a meal or while he is standing up. Emaciation becomes extreme and the patient cannot be roused from sleep. Death follows if other diseases, such as pneumonia or infection with other parasites, are not its direct cause.

The disease caused by *T. gambiense* and *T. rhodesiense*, namely, African trypanosomiasis, occurs in the parts of Africa in which the tsetse flies, which transmit these species of trypanosomes, occur. The area inhabited by the tsetse flies is enormous. It has been estimated that it covers about $4\frac{1}{2}$ million square miles, which is about 50 times the area of Great Britain. All the species of tsetse flies that transmit *T. gambiense* and *T. rhodesiense* do not, however, occur all over this area. Their distribution varies and they exist in regions called 'fly belts', which do not for long remain the same.

The lives of the flies are controlled by a number of climatic and other factors which are so complex that they cannot be discussed here. Important among them is the kind of food that these flies must have. Some species of tsetse flies live only on the blood of certain vertebrate hosts, so that they depend upon these hosts. *G. palpalis*, for example, which is one of the chief vectors of human trypanosomiasis in West Africa, feeds, not only on the blood of man, but also on the blood of crocodiles, lizards and amphibia that occur in the rivers and lakes that this species of tsetse fly frequents. *G. tachinoides*, on the other hand, usually lives away from human settlements and prefers the blood of wild game, such as antelope, and that of other animals that live in the rivers. Both these species, together with *G. pallidipes*, *G. fusca*, and *G. brevipalpis*, are among the species of tsetse flies that depend upon the shade and humidity that they find along the thickly-wooded shores of lakes and rivers. Usually they tend to travel up the rivers in the wet season and down them when the dry season comes, to the heavier bush found along the lower reaches of the rivers. These species, because they depend on the vegetation along these waterways, are called *riverine* species and usually they depend, not merely on the vegetation as such, but on the shade and humidity provided by certain kinds of vegetation. If these types of vegetation are removed by man, these species of tsetse flies cannot maintain themselves and this is, in fact, what is done. The clearing of the shores of rivers and lakes of the kind of vegetation favoured by the flies is one of the chief means employed in the control of tsetse flies.

Riverine species of tsetse flies of this kind may be contrasted with species of tsetse flies that are found, not typically along the shores of rivers and lakes, but in more open savannah country. These species are called *non-riverine* species. Examples of them are *G. morsitans*, *G. swynnertoni*, and *G. austeni*. They frequent, in these more open spaces, the shade of certain types of trees. Like the riverine species they show certain preferences for the blood of certain vertebrate hosts. *G. morsitans*, for instance, which is the most widely-distributed of all the species of tsetse flies, normally feeds on the blood of wild game, especially that of hoofed (ungulate) animals. For this reason they are often called 'game-flies'. *G. pallidipes* and *G. swynnertoni* are also game-flies that normally feed, not on man, but on wild game. *G. morsitans* and *G. pallidipes* usually feed on the blood of the wild pig.

Certain other features of the biology of the tsetse flies also tend to limit their geographical distribution. Tsetse flies do not lay eggs. Their larvae develop, one at a time, inside the womb (*uterus*) of the female fly, where they are nourished by 'milk glands', much as the young of human beings are. When they are mature, they are laid by the mother fly in warm moist soil, or under the bark of trees, or in other sheltered situations. The different species lay their larvae in different localities. Very soon each larva, if it is not killed by sunlight, which will readily kill it, or by some other external agency, becomes a pupa enclosed in a hard, protective case and, after about five weeks, the adult fly is ready to burst off the lid of the pupa case and begin its adult life. Each female produces only 12 to 14 larvae before she dies. As one entomologist has said, it is astonishing that tsetse flies, which produce so few young and are less numerous in Africa than other insects are, and depend upon certain degrees of temperature and humidity and on the shade of certain types of vegetation only, and also need, every three days or so, a meal of the blood of certain kinds of animals, survive the elaborate and costly attacks that man makes in his efforts to exterminate them from the world.

Tsetse flies are usually most active during the daylight

hours and feed more in the early morning and evening rather than in the heat of the day, when they seek the shade of the kind of vegetation that they prefer. They hunt by sight, and fly a few feet from the ground, buzzing as they go. Moving objects attract them and some non-riverine species, such as *Glossina morsitans*, will follow men and animals for considerable distances. They will also follow steamboats moving on the rivers. Riverine species like *G. palpalis*, however, do not usually travel far from the shores of lakes and rivers and they attack men and animals at fords and drinking places.

The measures taken by man to protect himself and other animals from the bites of the tsetse flies and to exterminate them, are expensive and laborious. They include the use of fly-screens applied to the doors and windows of houses or to vehicles, domesticated animals, and steamboats on the rivers; the wearing of white clothing, which tends to repel the flies, as white skins also do, the flies being more attracted to brown or black skins or to clothes of these darker colours; the spraying of fly-screens and cattle with DDT and the spraying of insecticides by means of aeroplanes over the habitats of the flies; the use of chemical substances that repel, to some extent at any rate, the flies; and such costly and elaborate measures as the removal of whole human communities, together with their domesticated animals, to areas that have been previously cleared of the flies or are, for other reasons, out of their reach. The social, administrative, and economic consequences of these removals of human communities are complex. They are complicated by such consequences as soil-erosion caused by over-population of the new areas colonized, by conflicts that develop with the traditional practices and the religion of the people removed, and by such problems as those that arise from the fact that domesticated animals are, to the African native, not only sources of food, but evidence of power and social position, or may be needed, whether they are in good condition or not, as bridal dowries or for religious ceremonies. Nevertheless, removals of large communities of natives have been successfully carried out. The Anchau Settlement in Nigeria, for example, involved an area of 7,000 square miles and in other parts of Africa similar operations of this kind have been successfully completed.

The measures taken to combat the flies themselves take advantage of the detailed knowledge of the biology of the flies that entomologists have laboriously gained. One of the earliest methods of attacking the flies, namely, catching the flies by hand, is used effectively in certain areas. Combined with the Symes block-method of clearing vegetation, it was, for example effective against *Glossina palpalis* along the shores of Lake Victoria and the rivers of Kenya and the southern Sudan. The Symes method clears blocks of riverine vegetation about two miles long and separates them by clearings about 1,000 yards wide. Paths are cut in the vegetation along river banks and lake shores, and people with nets patrol these on several days each week and catch as many flies as they can. In one block this method reduced the number of flies caught from 5,000 in three months in 1933 to seven in nine months in 1935, the cost being £40 a week, in contrast to £250 a mile needed for complete clearing of the vegetation.

Less effective against some species are traps designed to induce the female flies to deposit their larvae in places where the larvae and pupae can be destroyed; but traps have been effective against some species, such as *G. palpalis* and *G. pallidipes*. Cattle and other animals can be used as bait to attract the flies, which are then caught and killed, and this method is used for counting the numbers of flies in particular areas.

Another method used is the prohibition of the burning of grass, which is practised by native hunters. Burning the grass destroys seedlings and shoots and interferes with the natural succession of vegetation and the normal thickening of woodland. It may destroy ants that prey on the pupae of the tsetse flies. Prohibition of fires (*fire-exclusion*) retains, it is believed, the grass-covering of the land and allows a matt of grass to form which is disadvantageous to the pupae of the flies because it increases the moisture of the land; it may also prevent the production of larvae by the flies, because it increases the humidity of the air; it also encourages the ants that prey on the pupae and favours thickening of woodland. Fire-exclusion has been effective against such non-riverine species as *G. morsitans* and *G. swynnertoni* in Tanganyika, but in northern Nigeria, where it increased the density of woodland, it provided shelter for, and encouraged the survival of, *G. morsitans*.

The control or destruction of wild game is another method used to combat the tsetse flies. Its object is to remove the antelope, wild pig, and other animals on whose blood the tsetse flies feed. From these animals the flies may take up trypanosomes and transmit them to man and his domesticated stock. Destruction of game has been used chiefly to combat such non-riverine species as *G. morsitans* in Rhodesia and Bechuanaland. This species prefers the blood of wild game, and seems to be largely dependent on this, although it will take, when the blood of wild game is not available, the blood of domesticated stock, and, when this is also denied to it, human blood. It frequents hot, dry areas and retreats from human settlements. A settlement of 200 people per square mile may, in fact, drive *G. morsitans* away from man. In Rhodesia the efficiency of the destruction of wild game has certainly been proved. In 1939 it cleared the fly out of at least 6,000 square miles of the country and made it possible to open roads to transport pulled by oxen. In Tanganyika, on the other hand, experts doubt its efficacy. It has been argued that it cannot be sufficiently thorough, that it is especially difficult, if not impossible, to eradicate wild pig, that the wild game are not important reservoirs of the two species, *T. gambiense* or *T. rhodesiense*, that infect man and that game destruction is therefore chiefly valuable against trypanosomes that cause diseases of domesticated stock. This stock, it is argued, themselves so often harbour latent infections with trypanosomes from which healthy animals may be infected that it is useless to try to exterminate the wild game. There are also cogent humanitarian and aesthetic arguments against this method of control of trypanosomiasis.

Although all these methods of combating tsetse flies are useful, the most effective method of all is the clearing of the vegetation on which these flies depend for the shade and humidity that they must have. Removal of this vegetation may effectively prevent the spread of the flies and may defend man and his domesticated animals from them. Disadvantages of this method are its cost, and the labour and time required, but it can be combined with land reclamation and other measures which make it possible to colonise rich areas from which man would otherwise be debarred by the tsetse fly.

Clearing of vegetation is done by poisoning or ring-barking selected trees, or by felling and trimming them, or removing them by means of bull-dozers or other machines. Clearing which removes certain trees that are favoured by certain species of tsetse fly is called *selective clearing*. Complete or partial clearance of certain sites or the removal of certain types of vegetation from these areas is called *discriminative clearing*; this is useful against non-riverine species, such as *Glossina morsitans*, which shelters in open woodland and prefers moimbo or against *G. swynnertoni*, which likes thorn-bush. Against riverine species, such as *G. brevipalpis* and *G. pallidipes*, undergrowth is cut out, only large trees with clean stems being left. A clearing ten yards wide and a quarter of a mile long may thus be made. To combat *G. palpalis* all heavy forest and thicket must be removed and the clearings should extend for a quarter of a mile from cultivated land. In Nigeria the tributaries of the main rivers dry up in the dry season and the tsetse flies leave these tributaries for the lower reaches of the river, but may come back in the wet season. *Barrier clearings* can therefore be made to prevent their return and these have been successful features of the Anchau Settlement and other operations of the same kind. In the Gold Coast clearings, combined with mass treatment of the people with drugs that kill the trypansomes, have been very successful. In 1937, some 30,000 square miles of country were involved and 5 to 15 per cent of the people were infected with trypanosomes, the chief vectors being the riverine species *G. palpalis* and *G. tachinoides*. The disease caused depopulation of the area of the Black Volta River and its tributaries, and as a result the watersheds between the rivers became overcrowded and soil-erosion and land-hunger followed. The first attempts at control of the flies by means of clearings of the vegetation reduced the incidence of trypanosomiasis in five years by 60 to 80 per cent, but they did not bring about a progressive decline of the disease. It was then found that the flies were most vulnerable when they travelled down the rivers in the dry season and concentrated in limited areas lower down the waterways and selective clearings made in these areas, carried out in 1941–2 in the Lawra district, caused a rapid disappearance of dense colonies of *G. palpalis* and *G. tachinoides*. Selective clearing thus made it possible to return the people to good land and grazing in the river valleys.

Trypanosoma cruzi

This species, which causes the type of trypanosomiasis that attacks man, not in Africa, but in South America, differs considerably from the two species that cause this disease in Africa. First, it lives, in man and in its other vertebrate hosts, not in the plasma of the blood, and the other body-fluids inhabited by the trypanosomes that cause African trypanosomiasis, but inside the cells of certain organs of the body. It does appear in the blood in the early stages of the disease that it causes, but later it may be difficult to find it in the blood. It is, therefore, chiefly an *intracellular* parasite.

The forms of it found in the blood of man are about 20 micra long and they are either long and slender trypanosomes, or short and broad ones. The kinetoplast of the short form is very large. This species does not multiply in the blood. Every now and then it disappears from the blood and is then found inside certain cells of the internal organs. It is often found in the cells of the muscles of the heart, but it also lives inside certain phagocytic cells, called the cells of the reticulo-endothelial system, in the spleen, liver, lymphatic glands, and bone-marrow.

When they enter these cells the trypanosomes throw off the flagellum and undulating membrane and become small, ovoid forms, about 1·5 to 4 micra in diameter. These forms have a structure similar to that of species of the genus *Leishmania* described above and they are therefore called *leishmanial forms*. They multiply inside their host-cells by longitudinal division until they form groups inside the cells. Later they become elongated and each of them grows a short flagellum and an undulating membrane with a kinetoplast situated in front of the trophonucleus. They then resemble species of the genus *Crithidia* described above and they are called *crithidial* forms. These crithidial forms in their turn multiply by longitudinal division and finally become the trypanosome forms that are the only forms found in the blood that circulates at the periphery of the human body.

During this cycle therefore, this species of trypanosome assumes successively leishmanial, crithidial, and trypanosome

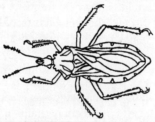

Fig. 46. An assassin bug (*Triatoma* sp.)

forms and thus shows, as the other species of the genus *Trypanosoma* do, the relationship between the three genera, *Leishmania*, *Crithidia*, and *Trypanosoma*.

The rest of the life history of *T. cruzi* occurs, in the course of six to fifteen days, in the food canal only of blood-sucking bugs (Hemiptera), belonging to the family Reduviidae (fig. 46). The species of these bugs which thus act as vectors of this species of trypanosome are *Panstrongylus* (*Triatoma*) *megistus*, *Panstrongylus geniculatus*, *Eutriatoma sordida*, *Triatoma infestans*, *Rhodnius prolixus*, and *Eratyrus cuspidatus*; but numerous other reduviid bugs have been found naturally infected with *Trypanosoma cruzi* and are therefore presumably able to transmit this trypanosome to man. Further a number of hard and soft ticks and the bed-bug, *Cimex lectularius*, can be experimentally infected with *Trypanosoma cruzi* and are therefore possibly able to infect man and other animals.

Because there are so many vectors of *Trypanosoma cruzi*, the chances of man becoming infected with it are greater than those of human infection with the two African species of human trypanosomes. The chances are all the greater because the incidence of this trypanosome in some species of the bugs, unlike that of the African species in the tsetse flies, may be as high as fifty per cent. The chances of human infection are also higher because *T. cruzi* has several normal hosts among the wild animals of South America. In this respect it resembles *Schistosoma japonicum* among the trematodes that infect man. *T. cruzi* may be present, for instance, in dogs, foxes, cats, armadillos, bats, opossums, anteaters, squirrels, and monkeys. Armadillos, which have a habit of burrowing down and coming up inside native huts, may be frequent sources of infection of the bugs that attack the inhabitants of the huts. This is, therefore, a species which has, not only many vectors, but many reservoir hosts.

In an insect vector the trypanosomes taken up from the blood of man or other vertebrate host pass to the middle part of the food canal of the bug and become crithidial forms. These multiply their numbers by longitudinal division and pass to the hinder part of the food canal, where leishmanial forms appear and these give origin to the metacyclic trypanosome forms which are the infective phases. How do these infective forms get from the food canal of the bugs into the blood of their vertebrate hosts? They cannot be inoculated through the skin of these hosts, because they do not pass, as the infective forms of the African trypanosomes do, into the vector's salivary glands. They are in the hinder part of the food canal of the bugs. But these bugs, when they suck the blood of man or other vertebrates, often pass out excreta on to the skin in the neighbourhood of the bite. The infective forms of the trypanosomes are in the excreta and, when the host rubs the area irritated by the bite of the bug, the infective forms of the trypanosomes are rubbed into the wound and thus get into the blood of the vertebrate host. Man and the other vertebrate hosts thus actually infect themselves with this species of trypanosome by an act of their own. This method of infection by contamination of a wound made by the vector with its infected excreta is called the *contaminative* method of infection. Another trypanosome that infects its vertebrate host in this

The Human Trypanosomes

manner is the harmless species, *Trypanosoma lewisi*, of the rat, the vector of which is rat-flea, *Nosopsyllus fasciatus*.

The reduviid bugs which transmit *T. cruzi* are active and bite chiefly during the night. They are often numerous in native huts and they bite people when they are asleep. They bite chiefly on the face and round the mouth and are, for this reason, called 'kissing bugs'.

The disease caused by *T. cruzi* is often called Chagas's disease, to commemorate the name of the Brazilian doctor, Carlos Chagas, who discovered that *T. cruzi* is the cause of it. It affects chiefly children younger than three years old, but it may attack older children and adults. It is, so far as we know, confined to South America and Mexico. It is commonest in Brazil, especially in the state of Minas Gerais, but it has more recently been found in Chile, northern Argentina, Bolivia, Peru, Ecuador, Venezuela, Columbia, Costa Rica, El Salvador, Guatemala, and in parts of Mexico.

Most often infection occurs through the mucous membranes in the regions of the outer angle of the eye and of the nostrils and lips. It is possible that the metacyclic trypanosomes can, under certain circumstances, actually penetrate through the intact skin. The metacyclic trypanosomes enter phagocytic cells in the skin and also the fat cells and muscle cells underlying the skin. Inside these cells they multiply and become trypanosome forms, which enter the blood and are distributed to various organs of the body, in which they continue to live. Often the infection causes no symptoms, but, if it does, the disease caused may be acute or chronic. First a local reaction occurs round the site of the infection, which is frequently round the mouth or eyes. A swelling occurs here or the eyelids of one eye swell up. Later in acute cases, fever, oedema, and anaemia develop and, because this species of trypanosome often shows a preference for the cells of the muscles of the heart, cardiac symptoms develop which may end in death. If the patient survives, the symptoms may disappear. The disease may, on the other hand, become chronic and the effects of the trypanosomes on the heart may cause weakness and degeneration of the heart muscle and ultimate death.

The Genus Leishmania

The species of this genus (figs. 42D, 47) are, like *Trypanosoma cruzi,* intracellular parasites. During most of their life histories they are found typically inside the phagocytic cells of various organs and they have the leishmanial structure described above. Each individual is, that is to say, a small, pear-shaped or oval organism 2 to 5 micra long by 1·5 to 2·5 micra

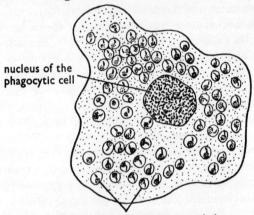

nucleus of the
phagocytic cell

leishmanias, each with a rounded
trophonucleus and a rod-shaped
kinetoplast

Fig. 47. *Leishmania tropica,* the cause of Oriental Sore (cf. fig. 42D). Several individuals inside a phagocytic cell of the human body

broad, inside which there is a trophonucleus and a kinetoplast. The flagellum and undulating membrane are absent from the individuals that live inside the cells, but a flagellum appears during the phase of the life history that occurs in the food canals of the sand flies that transmit them to man and other vertebrate hosts. Among these vertebrate hosts are man, the dog, some rodents, such as the gerbil, and some other mammals.

Inside the phagocytic cells of the vertebrate hosts the leishmanias multiply their numbers by longitudinal division, much as their relatives, the trypanosomes, do, and this multiplication often goes on till the host-cell is packed with the parasites.

It is, as yet, uncertain whether the leishmanias can leave the host-cell and enter other phagocytic cells. It seems probable that they are originally engulfed by these phagocytic cells, which may succeed in destroying some of them. At all events, when the vectors, which are always sand flies, suck the blood of man or the other invertebrate hosts, they take up the phagocytic cells containing the leishmanias and the leishmanias are not digested by the sand flies. They become, in the middle part of the food canal of the sand fly, forms which have the structure of species of the genus *Leptomonas* (fig. 42c), which are found in the food canals of fleas, horse flies, and some other insects and other animals, such as shell-fish, roundworms, and reptiles. They become, that is to say, elongated individuals with a flagellum at the anterior end, and in their bodies there is a trophonucleus and, near the origin of the flagellum, a basal granule and a kinetoplast. But there is no undulating membrane. The occurrence of these leptomonad forms in the life histories of species of the genus *Leishmania* indicates that *Leptomonas* is related to the genera *Trypanosoma, Crithidia* and *Leishmania*.

The leptomonad forms formed in this manner multiply their numbers rapidly till they fill the midgut of the sandfly. Some of them attach themselves, by means of their flagella, to the walls of the midgut; others lie free in its cavity. Later they spread forwards to the gullet (*oesophagus*) and pharynx and gradually block these up. When the sand fly now tries to suck the blood of man or any other vertebrate host, the plug of leptomonad forms of the leishmanias prevents the flow of blood. The sand fly still tries to get a meal of blood and, in its efforts to do this, some of the leptomonad forms of the leishmanias get through the sand fly's proboscis and are inoculated into the blood of the vertebrate host. It is possible, also, that if the leptomonad forms are ejected on to a wound or abrasion on the skin of the vertebrate host, they may be able to enter the vertebrate host through this. Once they are in the blood of the vertebrate host these leptomonad forms lose their flagella and become leishmanial forms and these are ingested by the phagocytic cells just under the skin of the vertebrate host.

The subsequent fate of the leishmanias depends on the

species of the genus *Leishmania* to which they belong. There are two species of this genus, *Leishmania tropica* and *Leishmania donovani*.

Leishmania tropica causes the disease called cutaneous leishmaniasis or Baghdad or tropical or Oriental sore. This species, as the name of the disease implies, does not spread beyond the skin of the vertebrate host. The leishmanias remain in the phagocytes of skin, where they cause the formation of ulcers which refuse to heal. This disease occurs in man and dogs in Southern China, north-east India, Arabia, Central Asia, the Caucasus, and all along the Mediterranean coasts of southern Europe and north Africa; it also occurs in New Mexico and pretty well all over South America. A form of it called espundia, which attacks man in central and South America, especially in the forests of Brazil and Peru, is characterized by the formation of ulcers of mucous membranes adjoining the skin, such as those of the mouth and naso-pharynx, which may spread and cause destruction of tissues and terrible deformation. Some experts think that the species of the genus *Leishmania* that causes this disease is a distinct species, to which they give the name *Leishmania brasiliensis*.

In central Asia Russian workers have found that *Leishmania tropica* naturally infects, in regions in which man is also infected, certain wild rodents, especially the sousliks and the gerbils, which develop typical sores on their ears; and that sand flies transmit infection with these species to these rodents. The sand flies follow these rodents into their burrows and maintain the infection in them, so that these rodents are reservoir hosts from which the sand flies communicate the disease to man when they leave the rodents and seek human blood.

Leishmania donovani, the other species of the genus *Leishmania*, does not remain in the skin. Phagocytes containing the parasites enter the blood and are carried by the blood to other organs of the body and the leishmanias become parasitic in these. The first sign of infection is a small papule on the skin which disappears, but later the parasites are found in the phagocytic cells in the liver, spleen, bone-marrow, lymph glands and the walls of the intestine, as well as in the phagocytic cells in the blood. The results of this general invasion of the body are at first headache, irregular fever, and enlargement of the spleen and later an irregular, undulant fever, anaemia, emaciation, diarrhoea, bleeding from the mucous membranes of the mouth and nose, and finally death. The incubation period extends from ten days to about a year, but is usually two to four months after infection. When the disease is acute it may kill the patient in a few weeks; but death may not occur for a year, or even, in chronic cases, two or three years. If the disease is not treated, 90 to 95 per cent of adult patients and 75 to 85 per

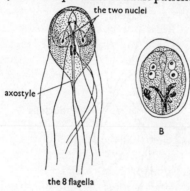

Fig. 48. *Giardia intestinalis.*
(A) trophozoite; (B) cyst

cent of infants die of it. Treatment with antimony preparations will cure 85 to 95 per cent of infected people.

Other Flagellates Parasitic in Man

Apart from the trypanosomes, which are extracellular parasites of the blood, and the leishmanias, which are intracellular parasites of the phagocytic cells, there are other species of flagellated Protozoa that are able to cause human disease. One of these lives in the food canal of man; the other lives in the vaginal canal of women. The two species are *Giardia (Lamblia) intestinalis*, which lives in the first part of the intestine (*duodenum*) and *Trichomonas vaginalis*, which occurs in the vaginal canal.

Giardia intestinalis (fig. 48) is a small flagellate, 10 to 18 micra long, which differs in structure from most other Protozoa, because it is bilaterally symmetrical and it has two sets of organs in its body. Its body is shaped like a pear flattened on its ventral side, on which there is a shallow depression, used by the parasite as a kind of sucker with which it adheres to the cells that line the duodenum. Inside the body there are two nuclei and other structures which need not concern us here; and the organism has the eight flagella shown in fig. 48A. With these flagella *Giardia* swims along more or less in a straight line,

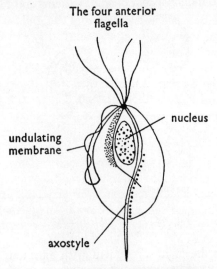

The four anterior flagella

nucleus

undulating membrane

axostyle

Fig. 49. *Trichomonas vaginalis*

its body swaying from side to side as it goes. It feeds by absorbing through its body surface nutritive materials in the contents of the host's food canal.

Its life history is simple and direct. In the human food canal it multiplies its numbers, sometimes with great rapidity, by dividing longitudinally. Its method of leaving one host to find another is to enclose itself in a protective cyst-wall (fig. 48B) and to pass out of the host in its excreta. These oval cysts, which are 10 to 14 micra long, get into the food or drink of other human beings, and thus infect them.

The Human Trypanosomes

Giardia intestinalis is common enough in man all over the world, though it is probably commoner in the warmer countries. Some 5 to 16 per cent of people examined have been found infected with it and it is especially common in children. Many quite healthy people harbour it in their food canals and do not suffer in any way, but, if any other condition upsets the processes of digestion, or sets up in the duodenum conditions favourable to the multiplication of the lamblias, these organisms multiply enormously and may then aggravate the condition. Some experts believe that they are, in any circumstances, liable to cause inflammation of the gall bladder or of the ducts which carry the bile to the intestine, but there is no conclusive proof of this.

Species of the genus *Giardia* are found in the food canals of many other vertebrate animals. One, for instance, is very common in the mouse. Others are found in the rat, the guinea pig, and the dog.

Trichomonas vaginalis

This species (fig. 49) is a pear-shaped organism about 13 micra long, which is found in the vagina of women all over the world. It is also found in the genito-urinary tract of men. It is commoner in women suffering from various forms of inflammation of the vagina and may be present in 70 per cent of women thus afflicted.

It has, as the figure shows, a flagellum that runs backwards down its body to a point about half-way to the posterior tip of the body and this flagellum is united to the body by an undulating membrane similar to the undulating membrane of a trypanosome. In other species of the genus *Trichomonas* this flagellum that runs backwards along the body continues right to the posterior end of the organism's body and may continue beyond this to become free in the fluid in which the organism lives.

In addition to this backwardly-directed flagellum, *Trichomonas vaginalis* has four other flagella, which arise from its anterior end and lash about freely in the fluid in which the *Trichomonas* lives. Down the middle of its body runs a stiff rod, called the *axostyle*, which projects beyond the posterior end of the body. Near the anterior end there is a slit-like mouth (*cytostome*), through which the organism takes in bacteria and food material present in the vaginal canal.

The life history of *Trichomonas vaginalis* is simpler even than that of *Giardia*. In the vagina it multiplies its numbers by longitudinal division; but it does not form cysts. It is unable to live outside the human body. It is supposed that it is transferred from one woman to another by the sexual act performed with men infected with it, but there is no proof of this and the exact method by which it is transferred is not known. Some experts think that it is a harmless organism and certainly many women harbour it without showing any symptoms of the infection. On the other hand some gynaecologists think that *Trichomonas vaginalis* causes a form of inflammation of the vagina and of other parts of the female genito-urinary system. One of its relatives, *Trichomonas foetus*, is a serious cause of abortion in cattle; but there is no evidence that *Trichomonas vaginalis* ever does this. Another of its relatives, *Trichomonas hominis*, lives in the large intestine of man, where it is a harmless commensal. *Trichomonas tenax*, another harmless commensal, lives in the human mouth and may be present in the mouths of healthy people as well as in those of people who have faulty teeth or disease of the mouth itself.

CHAPTER TEN

The Skin as a Home or a Source of Food

In this chapter we shall consider parasitic animals that live, not in the internal organs of the human body, but on its surface, or actually in the substance of the skin. Among these species are such insects as the fleas and lice and the maggots of other insects that may be parasitic in the skin; and, among the arachnids, the mites that cause scabies and similar diseases. The other species to be described are mostly such temporary parasites of man as the blood-sucking insects and ticks which feed upon his blood or other tissue fluids. Some of the blood-sucking insects have already been mentioned in earlier chapters – the mosquitoes, for instance, which transmit the malarial and filarial parasites, the tsetse flies and blood-sucking bugs which infect man with trypanosomes, the tabanid flies of the horsefly and cleg group, which carry to man the eyeworm and may, together with the stable fly, mechanically infect man and other animals with trypanosomes. There remain the leeches, which are, in some parts of the world, very annoying pests; and the blood-sucking bats.

THE LEECHES (HIRUDINEA)

The details of the anatomy of leeches need not concern us here. They are ringed worms (Annelida), related to the earthworm and the lugworm of our sea shores, but they are specially adapted for feeding on the blood of various animals. The crop, sometimes called the stomach, has numerous lateral offshoots in which the blood removed from the host can be stored, so that a leech can do without a meal of blood for a considerable time. Leeches have a sucker at the anterior end of the body round the mouth, and another at the posterior end. They can either swim in water or they can loop along, in water or out of it, by fixing one end of the body with one sucker and then stretching out the very extensible body to take hold with the other sucker, the sucker first fixed being then brought up to the second one. Some leeches were, as we all know, formerly used by doctors for removing blood from people who were ill and occasionally they are still used in this way. Leeches make, and inject into the host's blood, substances (*anticoagulins*) which delay the clotting of the blood, so that a good meal of blood is assured. It will be remembered that the hookworms and some other species of blood-sucking parasitic animals also do this.

The leeches that will feed on human blood belong to one only of the groups into which the leeches are divided, namely, the group called the Gnathobdellidae, which have three jaws beset with small teeth. The species formerly used for medicinal purposes are *Hirudo medicinalis* (fig. 2B), which was used in Britain; the species sometimes called the Algerian Dragon, *Hirudo troctina*; and the species used in Pakistan, *Gnathobdella ferox*. Other species not used medicinally may attack man in the tropics and these may cause, not only great annoyance, but anaemia due to loss of blood. These species are either terrestrial or aquatic.

The land leeches that attack man belong to the genus *Haemadipsa*. Typical of them is *Haemadipsa zeylanica*, a small leech, about 2 to 3 cm. ($\frac{3}{4}$ to $1\frac{1}{4}$ inch) long, which attacks man and other animals in Ceylon, India, and Malaya. It frequents trees, grass, and rank vegetation kept damp by tropical rains, or it lives under stones or other solid objects. It can force itself through human clothes, even penetrating, some observers record, the finest meshes of stockings, and it fastens itself on to the ankles or feet, or it may climb up the body inside the clothes, or attach itself to the throat. These leeches may be seen in the grass beside native paths, not idly waiting, but poised erect and ready to attack the passer-by. They are so small, and the wound they make causes so little irritation, that people attacked by them often do not know that the leeches are sucking blood, until bleeding from the part attacked tells them that this is so. The bare ankles of natives may be festooned with them. Horses may be driven wild by numbers of these leeches attached to their fetlocks and other animals also suffer. The points at which the leeches have fed go on bleeding after the leeches have dropped off, because the leeches have injected substances that prevent the clotting of the blood. Anaemia may therefore follow, or the bleeding points may become inflamed and may ulcerate. Some of the substances used to repel insects may prevent their attacks, or brine or vinegar may make them drop off the skin.

Another species of this genus, *Haemadipsa japonica*, which has similar habits, attacks man and other animals in Japan, the Philippine Islands, Java, Borneo, Sumatra, and southwest Asia generally; and three species, *H. fallax*, *H. morsitans*, and *H. vagans*, are similar pests in Madagascar. In southern Australia a land leech now placed in the genus *Philaemon* attacks man and there are other species that feed on human blood in Chile and Trinidad.

The aquatic leeches from which man may suffer cause more unpleasant symptoms. They are usually taken into the mouth accidentally when water is drunk, or they may get into the vagina of women or the urethra of men when they bathe. Several species of leeches have been reported from the interior of the body of man, but the species most often concerned is *Limnatis nilotica*. This species lives in streams and lakes and quiet waters in Southern Europe, the Mediterranean coast of northern Africa from Egypt to Morocco, the Canary Islands and Azores, and in western Asia from Palestine to the borders of India. Related species have been described from Singapore and India and, in Africa, from Senegal and the Congo River area.

A fully-grown *Limnatis nilotica* is 8 to 12 cm. (3 to $4\frac{3}{4}$ inches) long, but it is the younger, smaller leeches that may be accidentally taken into the human body. When they are taken in with drinking water the leeches may attach themselves to the mucous membrane of the throat, nose, epiglottis, or the gullet; or they may be drawn by breathing into the larynx, or into the breathing tubes of the lungs. Their jaws are too weak to penetrate human skin, but they can attach themselves to the softer mucous membranes and suck blood. The actual bite causes little pain, but the leeches secrete substances that prevent the clotting of the blood, so that bleeding may go on for some time and progressive anaemia may result and death has been attributed to this. There may also be other symptoms, which vary according to the position occupied by the leech, such as feelings of pressure, coughing, difficulty in swallowing, pain in the chest, loss of speech, or even suffocation. *Limnatis nilotica* was, it is said, a troublesome pest of French troops in Egypt many years ago.

THE BLOOD-SUCKING BATS

Much has been written in the past about the blood-sucking habits of various species of bats, but it is now known that few of them normally suck human blood. The vampire bat, *Vampyrella spectrum*, formerly regarded as being one of the horrors with which man is plagued, feeds, it is now known, mainly upon fruit. But one species of one genus of bats, the genus *Desmodus*, and species of the genera *Diphylla* and *Diaemus*, undoubtedly suck blood. They are all found in Brazil and other parts of tropical America. Species of the genera *Diphylla* and *Diaemus* are rare, but species of the genus *Desmodus* are remarkably cunning pests of man, cattle, horses, poultry, and other animals. They have large incisor teeth with sharp edges and with these they make a shallow, clean-cut scoop from the flesh, which goes on bleeding longer than a puncture does. This compensates these bats for their lack of substances that prevent the coagulation of the blood which are injected into the host by leeches, hookworms, and some other species that feed on blood. The stomach of species of the genus *Desmodus* is, like that of the blood-sucking leeches, adapted to take in a large store of blood. It has, instead of the lateral extensions that the stomachs of leeches have, a long tube-like extension in which the blood is stored. Bats of this genus show remarkable cunning in their search for blood. They steal on their victims at night when they are asleep, walking or sidling up to them and scooping out a piece of flesh so delicately that the victim does not waken up and is often not aware of the attack till bleeding wounds are discovered when the victim wakes up. The habits of these bats are well described by Allen (1940).

INSECTS, TICKS, AND MITES

The other parasitic animals that live either on the human skin, or in its substance, are all either insects or arachnids. The species that are insects are either lice or fleas and those that are arachnids are either ticks, mites, or the degenerate arthropods with wormlike bodies called the pentastomids.

With the exception of the pentastomids, all the insects and arachnids considered in this book visit the skin of man in order to suck blood or other tissue fluids and for this reason the organs around the mouth (mouthparts) with which they obtain this kind of food have been modified for piercing the skin of the host and for sucking up the fluid food. In different species of bloodsucking arthropods these modifications take different forms. It is not necessary in this book to describe all these different modifications in detail, but a brief description of the mouthparts of mosquitoes, tabanid flies, and tsetse flies may help the reader. They are best understood if we first briefly consider the mouthparts of an insect, such as the cockroach, whose mouthparts are adapted for chewing solid food.

The mouthparts of the cockroach (fig. 50) are, from above downwards:

1. An upper lip or *labrum*, above the mouth;
2. a pair of toothed mandibles, on each side of the mouth;
3. a pair of first maxillae, beside the mouth, each provided with a sensory palp;
4. a lower lip or *labium*, below the mouth, composed of a pair of second maxillae fused together, each second maxilla bearing a sensory palp.

The mouthparts of a mosquito (fig. 51) are elongated to form a piercing proboscis. The elongated upper lip is fused with another structure to form a combined structure called the

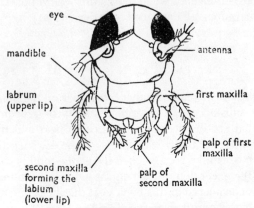

Fig. 50. Mouthparts of the cockroach
(*Periplaneta* sp.)

labrum-epipharynx, which forms a roof over the proboscis-tube; it is curved over at the sides, so that it has the form of a

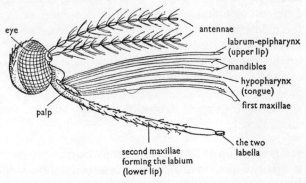

Fig. 51. Mouthparts of a female mosquito (*Culex* sp.)

tube incomplete below and it has been aptly compared to the outer cover of a bicycle or motor tyre. The floor of the incomplete tube thus formed is supplied by another elongate

structure called the *hypopharynx* or tongue. These two structures thus make up a tube through which the blood of the host
is sucked in. The skin of the host is pierced by the elongated
mandibles and first maxillae, which are modified to form delicate, piercing stylets. The tube formed by the hypopharynx
and labrum-epipharynx is then thrust into the wound. The
lower lip (*labium*), formed by the second maxillae, is an elongated, grooved structure in which the other mouthparts lie
when they are not in use. Hinged on to the free end of the
labium there are two flaps called the *labella* and, when the mosquito sucks blood, the piercing mouthparts are guided into the

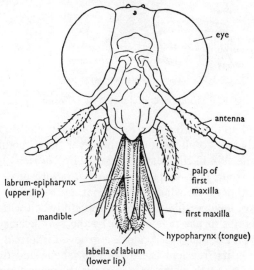

Fig. 52. Mouthparts of a tabanid fly

wound between these two labella, much as the cue of a billiards
player is guided between his thumb and forefinger (fig. 40).
As the piercing mouthparts sink into the wound made, the
labium is bent downwards to form a loop.

The mouthparts of a tabanid fly (fig. 52), such as a horse
fly, consist of the same elements, but the piercing mandibles
and maxillae are shorter and coarser and they move laterally
in the wounds. They therefore inflict more irritating bites. The

217

blood of the host is again sucked up in a tube formed by the labrum-epipharynx above and the hypopharynx below, but these flies can also suck up blood or other fluids along channels in the surface of the labella at the end of the lower lip.

The tsetse flies (fig. 53), like the stable fly, *Stomoxys calcitrans*, and the house flies and bluebottles and their relatives, have lost the mandibles and first maxillae. Blood is, however,

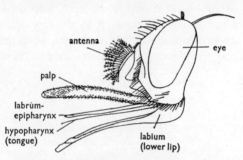

antenna

eye

palp

labrum-epipharynx

hypopharynx
(tongue)

labium
(lower lip)

Fig. 53. Mouthparts of a tsetse fly (*Glossina* sp.)

still sucked up through a tube formed by the upper lip and the tongue; these two elements are, however, now modified for piercing the skin of the host. The lower lip (*labrum*) has now become a stout, club-shaped, grooved structure in which the other mouthparts lie when they are not in use. It can be seen as a strong, bayonet-like structure held stiffly below the head; when it is not in use it is clothed by the two sensory palps, which lie on each side of it and are grooved internally to enclose it. On its free end there are two labella and these are provided with teeth which help to make the wound in the skin of the host. The mouthparts of the stable fly, *Stomoxys calcitrans*, are similar, but the lower lip is not enclosed by the palps.

The mouthparts of the fleas are shown in figs. 56, 57 and they need not be further described. The mouthparts of the sucking lice are tiny stylets enclosed in a sac beneath the head.

The mouthparts of all the arachnida (fig. 54) are altogether different from those of any insect. Arachnids are carnivorous creatures with very narrow mouths and they either suck up the blood and other tissue fluids of their prey after they have killed or paralysed it by injecting into it a poison made by their poison glands, or they kill or paralyse it and then tear it into small pieces. The head is absent from all arachnids, so that the feelers (*antennae*) present on the heads of other arthropods are also absent. Arachnids have, moreover, only two pairs of mouthparts, although the bases of the walking legs immediately behind the mouthparts may be used by some species as

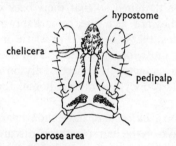

Fig. 54. Mouthparts of a hard tick (*Ixodes ricinus*)

accessory organs for tearing up or chewing the food. The two pairs of mouthparts are:

1. the *chelicerae*, which are used for grasping, holding, or crushing the prey or they may be modified to form pincers. In the parasitic ticks and mites they are modified for piercing the skin of a plant or animal host. In the spiders they contain the poison glands and end as claws or fangs.
2. The *pedipalps*, which are, in some species, sensory or stridulating organs, but are, in most arachnids, organs for dealing with the food. They may be, as they are in the scorpion, for example, large pincers used for catching and holding the prey. In the parasitic ticks and mites (Order Acarina), and only in this Order, the chelicerae and pedipalps are carried on a chitinous plate, called the *capitulum*, situated at the anterior end of the body, and this plate also bears a median, unpaired structure, called the *hypostome* (fig. 54), which is covered with teeth that project backwards. The pedipalps are, in these species, sensory organs and the chelicerae make

a way through the skin of the host, through which the hypostome is also thrust. The function of the hypostome is to hold on to the host and its recurved teeth prevent it from being pulled out.

The Lice

The lice (Order Phthiraptera) are wingless insects (Plate 5a,) with their bodies flattened so that their back comes near to their belly, and they are, as a rule, remarkably specific to their hosts. Each species, that is to say, is parasitic on only one kind of animal, or, at most, on only a few. The lice of poultry or cattle, for instance, cannot live successfully on man and those of sheep or cattle cannot live on the horse. Lice are divided into two groups.

One group, the *Mallophaga*, have mouthparts adapted for chewing. They live on the hairs, feathers, discarded cells of the surface layers of the skin, or other epithelial debris found on the skin. These species are often called biting lice, but this name is misleading, because most of them do not bite into their host's skin, although some of them puncture it and draw blood on which they feed. A better name for the Mallophaga is the chewing lice. Most of them are parasitic on birds and they are, for this reason, often called bird-lice; but this name also is misleading, because some of them, such as the common louse of the dog, *Trichodectes canis*, are parasitic on mammalian hosts.

The other group is the sucking lice (*Anoplura*), all of which feed exclusively on the blood or other tissue fluids of the host's body, which they suck after they have punctured the skin with the minute stylets in their mouths.

All lice, whether they are chewing or sucking lice, have, in addition to the flattening of the body which helps them to run about on their six legs on the surface of the host and to evade capture by the host, curved claws on the ends of their legs with which they can hold on to the hairs or feathers of the host. All lice pass all their life histories on the surface of the host and they cannot live long away from a host. They attach their eggs, called *nits* (Plate 5b), to the hairs or feathers of the host and the young that emerge from the eggs are like the parents. There is, that is to say, no metamorphosis. The nymph leaves the egg and after a series of moults on its skin, becomes the adult male or female louse.

Man is, fortunately for him, afflicted only by two species of lice. These are *Pediculus humanus* (Plate 5a), strains of which live either on the head (*P. humanus capitis*) or on the body (*P. humanus corporis*), and *Phthirus pubis*, the crab louse, which lives in the hair on the lower part of the abdomen (*pubis*) of man.

Pediculus humanus, the human body louse, is relatively large. The male is 2 to 3 mm. ($\frac{1}{12}$ to $\frac{1}{8}$ inch) long and the female a little larger; the males and females of the head louse are about half this size. In both the head and body louse the head is diamond-shaped and it bears a pair of dark-coloured, simple eyes, in front of which are a pair of feelers (*antennae*), each consisting of five pieces. The body is greyish-white. The three segments of the thorax are immovably fixed together, as they are in all sucking lice, and the flattened abdomen, behind the thorax, has nine segments, only seven of which are visible externally. At the sides of each abdominal segment there are dark-coloured thickenings of the horny (chitinous) covering of the body, called *paratergal plates* and, also at the sides of the abdominal segments, on the dorsal side, there are six pairs of openings (*spiracles*) into the breathing tubes (*tracheae*). Another pair of spiracles opens on the dorsal side of the middle segment of the thorax (*mesothorax*). The six pairs of strong legs are approximately equal in size and each bears a single claw.

Phthirus pubis is smaller than the head and body louse. The females are 0·8 to 1 mm. (up to $\frac{1}{25}$ inch) long, the males being smaller. The greyish-white body is less elongated and the head is more rectangular. The abdomen is relatively short and its segments are not so distinct, but the claws on the legs are relatively large and heavy.

The eggs of *Pediculus humanus* and *Phthirus pubis* are whitish objects about 0·8 mm. long. The head louse and the crab louse attach their eggs to the hairs of the head or the pubis by means of a material resembling chitin. The body louse attaches them to the fibres of the clothes, especially in folds or creases of these, or to blankets or other parts of the bedding. The eggs are not set upon stalks as those of the warble flies are. At the free end of each egg of *P. humanus* (Plate 5b, fig. 2), there is a lid (*operculum*), on which there are 15 to 20 tubercles on each of which there is an opening leading into an air-chamber, which communicates with the interior of the egg through a small pore. The first nymph which develops inside the egg is thus provided with air for breathing. Each female head louse may lay about 80 to 100 eggs during her lifetime, but the female body louse lays about 200 to 300, averaging 8 to 10 a day when she is in full egg-production. The crab louse, on the other hand, lays only about 50 eggs. The number of eggs laid varies according to the temperature and the supply of food.

The life histories of the body louse, the head louse, and the crab louse are simple and similar. The eggs hatch in 8 to 11 days according to the temperature and liberate a nymph, which resembles the adult. The nymph grows and moults its skin 3 times in about 2 weeks, when it becomes the adult louse. The average duration of the life history of *Pediculus humanus* is 12 to 18 days and that of *Phthirus pubis* about 15 days. It has been estimated that the female body louse lives 34 to 46 days, the female head louse 27 to 38 days and the female crab louse about 35 days. The males do not live so long.

Both the young and the adult lice suck human blood and reddened, elevated papules appear at the sites of their bites, but people who acquire some immunity to them may suffer little. Scratching of the bites in response to the irritation that they cause may result in sores which may become infected with bacteria. The irritation caused is most severe at night and it may deprive the infected individual of sleep, with the consequence that mental depression may be one of the symptoms. Older people suffer more than the young do. The body louse is an important vector of the organisms that cause endemic typhus fever, trench fever, and European relapsing fever. The head louse also spreads these diseases to a less extent, but the crab louse does not. Endemic typhus occurs in people confined in unhygienic and crowded prisons, or in armies, or among peoples suffering from famine. The lice readily spread under these conditions from one person to another and transmit the causative organism of the disease as they do so. Man is usually infected, not by the bite of an infected louse, but by rubbing the excreta of infected lice, or their dead bodies after they have been killed by the organism that causes endemic typhus, into the bite of the louse or into an abrasion on the skin. He is infected, that is to say, much as he is infected by *Trypanosoma cruzi*. He infects himself with the spirochaete that causes European relapsing fever in the same way. Trench fever is, however, transmitted either in this manner or by the bite of the louse.

THE FLEAS

The structure of a typical flea is shown in Plate 6; and the features of fleas that are, for one reason or another, important to man are shown in figs. 55 to 59.

The adaptations that fleas show to life on the surfaces of their hosts are different from those of lice. Their bodies are flattened, not from the back to the belly, but from side to side, and their legs, especially the third pair, are adapted to enable them to leap in the well-known manner that is one of their characteristics. Their powers of leaping help them to get from host to host and they are remarkable. Thus *Pulex irritans*, one of the fleas that attack man, may leap for a distance of 13 inches and to a height of nearly 8 inches. Each leg has a pair of claws that enable the flea to hold on to its host. The head is attached to the thorax without an intervening neck and it bears, in some species, a pair of coloured, simple eyes. The antennae are short and are usually held in grooves (*antennal grooves*) on the side of the head, though they can be erected out of these. On the lower, lateral border of the head, in the region of insects called the cheek or *gena*, there is, in some species of fleas, a row of strong, pigmented spines, which together make up a structure called the *genal comb* (*genal ctenidium*). In some species there is also a similar comb, the *pronotal comb* (*pronotal ctenidium*) on the posterior border of the first segment of the thorax. It is said that these combs help the fleas to move through the hairs or feathers of their bird or mammalian hosts. The mouth is provided with stylets that are not dissimilar from those of the mosquitoes and their relatives, but they are shorter. They are shown, together with names given to them, in figs. 56 and 57. Fleas feed exclusively on the blood of their hosts, but they can live for many days without a meal

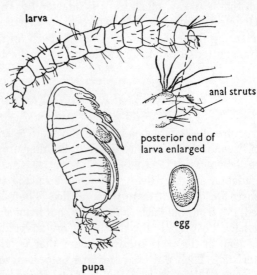

Fig. 55. Life history of a flea, showing the egg, larva and pupa, beneath which is the skin of the last larval stage

of blood. It was found, for instance, that *Pulex irritans* can live for 125 days without blood.

The three segments of the thorax are to some extent movable on each other. The abdomen has 10 segments and the 9th segment, in both male and female fleas, has, on its dorsal side, a sensory plate, provided with sensory hairs, which is called the *sensilium* (*pygidium*). It looks rather like a pin-cushion beset with pins. It has been suggested that it detects air currents, but its function is not exactly known. The dorsal side of the 9th segment of the male is modified to form a *clasper* with which the male holds the female during the sexual act and the penis of the male is a very complex structure that may be seen coiled inside the abdomen. The female has no claspers, but she can be recognized by the receptacle (*receptaculum seminis*) into which the sperms of the male are received.

Fleas, unlike lice, do not live all their life histories on the surfaces of their hosts. Only the adults live on the hosts; the rest of the life history occurs away from it. The oval, whitish, glistening eggs (fig. 55) are relatively large and may be 5 mm. ($\frac{1}{5}$ inch) long. They are rarely laid on the host. Usually they are laid in the crevices of floors of buildings in which the hosts live. The female flea may lay 3 to 18 eggs at a time and the female of one of the human fleas, *Pulex irritans*, may lay some 400 eggs in the course of her life, which may last about a year, although *Pulex irritans*, is known to have lived 513 days.

The fleas, unlike the lice, undergo a metamorphosis during their life histories. Inside the egg a first larva develops and this emerges from the egg by bursting the egg by means of a spine on its head. This larva (fig. 55) has no legs. It is yellow-ish-white and has two short antennae on its head, a thorax of three segments, and an abdomen of ten segments. On each of the thoracic and abdominal segments there are hairs and the last abdominal segment bears a pair of short, blunt, hooked processes, called the *anal struts*, with which the larva holds on to solid objects. These larvae are found in the crevices of floors and in the dust on them, under carpets and in similar places. They need moisture, but little food. They may eat blood in the excreta of adult fleas, but they do not suck blood from any host. Before they become mature the larvae moult their skins twice. Normally they are mature in 9 to 15 days, but unfavourable conditions may delay their development for as long as 200 days. The mature larva spins a whitish cocoon, inside which it becomes a pupa or chrysalis (fig. 55). The pupa is not enclosed in a protective membrane and its structure can be readily seen. The pupal stage may last for periods ranging from 7 days to a year, according to the external conditions to which it is exposed.

Another feature of fleas that differentiates them from lice is the fact that they do not restrict themselves to certain hosts

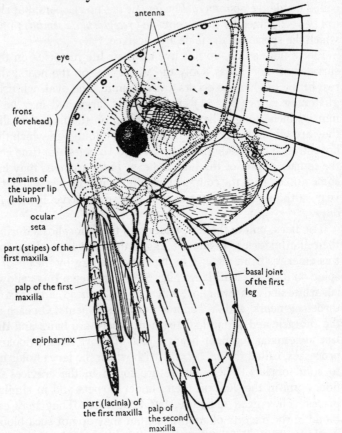

Fig. 56. Head of the human flea (*Pulex irritans*), showing the mouthparts and the absence of combs

only, as the lice do. Consequently man, and other hosts, may be attacked by several species of fleas. The species that are most often associated with man are:

Pulex irritans (fig. 56), often called the human flea, which is the commonest flea found on man in Europe and the western United States. Its hosts are dogs, rats, mice and other rodents and cattle and pigs and the badger.

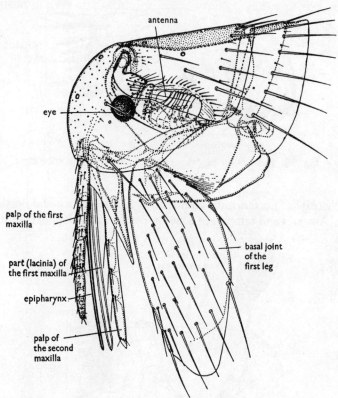

Fig. 57. Head of the plague flea (*Xenopsylla cheopis*), showing the mouthparts and the absence of combs

Xenopsylla cheopis (fig. 57), the Indian rat flea, which is common on rats in the tropics and subtropics. This is the flea most often associated with the transmission of bubonic plague to man. It will feed on mammals other than man and the rat.

Ceratophyllus gallinae (fig. 59), the common flea of the hen in Europe and the eastern United States. It readily bites man.

Ctenocephalides canis (fig. 58), the dog flea, and *Ctenocephalides felis*, the cat flea (Plate 6), both of which occur on dogs and cats all over the world.

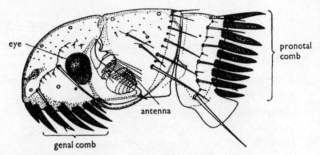

Fig. 58. Head of the dog flea (*Ctenocephalides canis*), showing the genal and ctenidial combs

Nosopsyllus fasciatus, the common rat flea of Europe and north America and temperate zones generally. Its chief host is the

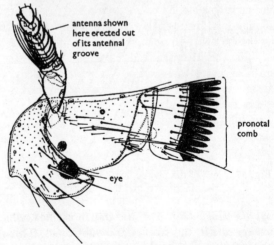

Fig. 59. Head of the hen flea (*Ceratophyllus gallinae*). This flea has a ctenidial comb, but no genal comb

brown rat, *Rattus norvegicus*. It transmits *Trypanosoma lewisi* to rats.

The Skin as a Home or a Source of Food

Leptopsylla segnis, a species common on the house mouse, and also on the rat and other small rodents.

Certain other species parasitic on squirrels and their relatives in the United States may also attack man.

In addition to these species there are two others which, because they have unusual habits, will be described separately below. These two species are:

Echidnophaga gallinacea, the stick-tight flea, which is a parasite of poultry in the tropics and subtropics. It also attacks man, dogs, cats, and birds other than the hen. The female burrows into the region of the head; and *Tunga penetrans*, the chigger or chigoe flea of tropical America and Africa, the female of which burrows into the skin of man, frequently between the toes.

The general effects of fleas are irritation caused by their bites. Reddened papules appear at the sites of the bites and these may, in some persons, be surrounded by swellings which cause considerable discomfort. Other persons, for reasons that are unknown, suffer little more than a transient itching of the area bitten. More important than the bites of fleas are the diseases that they may transmit to man. The two most important human diseases transmitted to man by fleas are bubonic plague and endemic (murine) typhus, both of which are diseases of rats.

Bubonic plague, caused by the bacillus *Pasteurella pestis*, is a disease of wild rodents that kills many of these hosts. Usually epidemics of plague follow epidemics among house rats that kill so many of the rats that the rat fleas seek the blood of man instead. The most important of the fleas that do this is *Xenopsylla cheopis*, which remains infective for a long time and is widely distributed, but *Xenopsylla astia* is a less important vector of plague in China and *Xenopsylla braziliensis* is a vector in East Africa. These fleas take up the plague bacilli and the bacilli multiply inside the digestive tract of the flea till it is blocked by masses of the bacilli and the fleas cannot suck blood. Such fleas are called 'blocked fleas'. They try persistently to suck blood and their efforts to do this cause regurgitation of the plague bacilli into the blood of man. Plague bacilli may be transmitted to man also by *Nosopsyllus fasciatus, Leptopsylla segnis*, and other species, but these species are less important. *Pulex irritans* can also transmit plague from rats to man and from man to man.

Endemic (murine) typhus, which must not be confused with epidemic typhus or with typhoid fever, is also a disease of rats that is transmitted from rat to rat and from rat to man by fleas. The most important vectors of it are *Xenopsylla cheopis, X. astia*, and *Nosopsyllus fasciatus*, but various other fleas, including the dog flea (*Ctenocephalides canis*), the cat flea (*Ctenocephalides felis*), and the stick-tight flea (*Echidnophaga gallinacea*) have been found naturally infected and may therefore be, at times, vectors.

Another disease that may be transmitted by fleas is tularaemia and fleas may transmit to man and other animals the organisms that cause anthrax and also other organisms that cause disease, which may be present in the droppings of the fleas. These infected droppings may be rubbed into the skin when the irritated area bitten by the fleas is rubbed or scratched. The dog flea (*Ctenocephalides canis*), and the cat flea (*Ctenocephalides felis*), and the human flea (*Pulex irritans*) are all intermediate hosts of the tapeworm of the dog, *Dipylidium caninum*, which may, as is explained in Chapter 6, be parasitic in man, especially in children; and the larvae of the rat flea, *Nosopsyllus fasciatus*, and those of *Xenopsylla cheopis* are among the intermediate hosts of the dwarf tapeworm, *Hymenolepis nana*, and of its relative, *H. diminuta*, both of which are described in chapter 6.

FLEAS THAT BURROW IN THE SKIN OF MAN

The Stick-Tight Flea (*Echidnophaga gallinacea*)

This species, which may be a dangerous pest of poultry, also attacks other birds and also, among mammals, dogs, cats, horses, rabbits, rats, and man. The adults are active, but during copulation the female flea attaches herself to the skin of the host and then burrows into the skin, forming a swelling which may ulcerate. In the lesion thus produced the female flea lays her eggs. The eggs drop down to the ground, where the larvae develop, as those of other fleas do. They become adult fleas in about a month.

The Chigoe or Chigger Flea (*Tunga penetrans*)

This species, which is also called the jigger or sand flea, inspired, according to Chandler (1955), the exclamation 'I'll be jiggered!' It is a small flea, about 1 mm. long, which attacks man, pigs, dogs, cats, and rats, in tropical America and Africa. It breeds especially in sandy, shaded soil or on the earthen floors of native huts and the adults attack the feet especially of man and animals. The females burrow into the skin, especially under the toe-nails, and live on the blood of the host. They produce eggs and retain them in their bodies, which swell up until they may be as large as a pea, the head and legs being then small appendages on the swollen body. The skin around the embedded flea becomes swollen and inflamed and painful and the two hindermost segments of the flea project from it. Through this protrusion the eggs are expelled to develop and produce larvae on the ground. The larvae spin a cocoon and pupate in this and the adults emerge from the pupa after about seventeen days or so.

The sites occupied by the burrowing female fleas may become very much inflamed and painful, especially if the flea is crushed and the eggs are set free into the skin. Expulsion of the flea leaves behind a sore that may become infected with bacteria and, if these bacteria get into the blood, blood-poisoning may result and it may be necessary to remove a toe or even a whole leg; or, if tetanus bacilli get into the wound, death may follow. Usually only a few chigger fleas infect an individual at one time, but some people may acquire heavy infections on the feet and other parts of the body.

THE BLOOD-SUCKING BUGS

The insects that the entomologist calls bugs belong to the Order of insects called the Hemiptera, all of which feed on the

231

tissue-fluids of either animals or plants, which they suck in after piercing the surface of the plant or animal host with a proboscis adapted for this purpose. Usually it can be seen folded back beneath the head. Some species of them are serious pests of crops and some transmit viruses to plants which cause serious plant diseases. The bugs are divided into two groups, the Homoptera and the Heteroptera, which are distinguished, as their names imply, by their wings. The Homoptera are not parasitic on man or other animals. They attack many of his cultivated plants. They have membraneous and often delicate wings that are held sloping over the body like the roof of a house. This large group includes the Cicadas, one of which occurs in Britain in the New Forest, the frog-hopper and cuckoo-spit insects, the tree-hoppers and leaf-hoppers, the species called plant-lice, examples of which are the apple-sucker and the pear-sucker which are very injurious to apples, the white flies that damage tomatoes and cucumbers grown in greenhouses, the scale-insects that injure various fruit plants, and the green-flies (aphids) which are pests of fruit trees, the grape vine and other plants.

The Heteroptera have wings the anterior portions of which are thickened and often sculptured and coloured and they lie flat on the body of the insect. This group includes the shield bugs, the lace bugs, the squash bug of North America which is a pest of cucurbitaceous plants, the American cinch bug, which destroys grasses and cereals, the Egyptian cotton-stainer bug, which damages cotton crops, the capsid bugs which attack apple and other fruit plants and also tea in Assam, and the pond-skaters that move about on the surfaces of ponds and streams, and the water-boatmen that swim in the water in these. To this group belong also the winged assassin or kissing bugs (fig. 46) (Reduviidae), mentioned in chapter 9 as vectors of *Trypanosoma cruzi* in South America, and the wingless bed bugs.

The bed bugs belong to the family Cimicidae. Species of this family have ovoid, flattened bodies with at most only traces of wings. The two species that most often attack man and other animals and suck their blood are: *Cimex lectularius* (fig. 60), which is prevalent in Europe and North America and temperate parts of the world generally; this species also feeds on poultry, doves, rats, mice, dogs, and cats; and *Cimex hemipterus*, which attacks man and other animals in India, Africa, and tropical parts of the world. In West Africa a species with longer legs, called *Leptocimex boueti*, also attacks man. Man may also be attacked at times by species of the genus *Cimex* which normally feed on the blood of pigeons and bats or

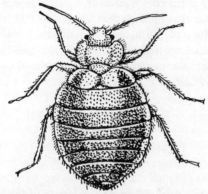

Fig. 60. The bed bug (*Cimex lectularius*)

by other species that feed on the blood of swallows or, in Mexico, poultry.

Bed bugs usually feed at night and hide by day in cracks and crevices in buildings, or in wooden bedsteads, under the wallpaper, and similar places. They need about fifteen minutes to take a full meal of blood and they feed every two days or so. They can live for as long as a year without a meal of blood. In cold weather they hibernate and do not feed.

The life history does not include a metamorphosis. The pearly-white, oval eggs are about 1 mm. long and the female bug lays 100 to 250 eggs during her life. In warm weather the eggs hatch in six to ten days and liberate a nymph that resembles the parent. This nymph moults its skin five times before the adult stage is reached and takes a meal of blood before each moult. If conditions are favourable, the adult stage is reached in seven to ten weeks. There may be three or four

generations of bugs in a year and the adults may live for as long
as a year or longer.

The bites of bed bugs may cause, in some individuals, considerable irritation and loss of sleep. If the bites are numerous
and go on for some time, anaemia and other symptoms may
result. In other individuals varying degrees of immunity to
the bites may be developed. Although the bed bug has naturally been suspected of transmitting a number of diseases to
man, including plague, kala-azar, typhus, leprosy, and yellow
fever, there is no evidence that it does, in fact, transmit these
diseases. Most of the attempts made to transmit these and
other diseases experimentally have failed. Bed bugs are therefore much less dangerous to man than the fleas, blood-sucking flies, and ticks that suck his blood.

HOUSEFLIES, BLOWFLIES, AND WARBLE FLIES

Man is unhappily able to provide, as sheep, cattle, and other
mammals are, attractive food for the young stages of insects
whose larvae normally live on decaying or putrefying vegetable materials, or develop, as the larvae of the warble flies of
cattle do, in the bodies of their hosts. The adult stages of these
insects are not parasitic. They visit man and other animals
only to lay their eggs on the surfaces of mammals, in situations
where the young that hatch out of the eggs can find suitable
food. The insects that do this are all insects with one pair of
wings only, which belong to the Order of insects called the
Diptera, as the tsetse flies and the stable fly also do. But the
insects that we are now considering are either relatives of the
house flies and the bluebottles or of the warble flies of cattle.

The house flies and their relatives spread to man and other
animals the organisms that cause a wide variety of diseases.
This they do, either because they carry bacteria on their feet
and deposit them on human food, or because they feed on decaying matter and other sources of infection and then feed on
sugar or other human foods or drinks and transmit the bacteria to these. Typhoid fever, typhus, cholera, tuberculosis, tu-
taraemia, anthrax, spirochaetes, organisms that cause inflam-

mation of the eyes, and even, in certain circumstances, certain trypanosomes and leishmaniasis, may all be conveyed mechanically to man by these flies. They may also suck up the cysts of *Entamoeba histolytica* from human excreta and thus spread amoebic dysentery and the eggs of some tapeworms and roundworms may be spread in the same way. These flies do not, however, act as true intermediate hosts of species parasitic in man. The maggots of house flies, however, may accidentally get into the intestine or even the urinary passages of man and may be found there. The larvae of bluebottles, flesh flies and other relatives of the house flies may also be found in the intestine of man.

The blowflies, however, and their relatives, the flesh flies and related species, are chiefly important because their young stages may become parasitic in the skin of man. They cause then the disease called *myiasis*, a term which is sometimes nowadays used to include any disease caused by a parasitic animal that lives in the skin or just under it; but it is, perhaps better to use this term only for diseases caused by the young of insects that live in the skin. An example of a myiasis caused by the maggots of an insect is the disease of sheep called strike, which will be well-known to many readers. This disease is caused by the maggots of blowflies which emerge from eggs laid on the skin of sheep, or in the wool, and feed on the tissues of the skin of the sheep, causing as they do this extensive and often fatal injuries.

Man, in the tropics and elsewhere, may be the victim of a similar disease. Various flies, the adults of which are always attracted by the odours of decaying flesh or vegetable matter, or by open, festering wounds, lay their eggs in material of this kind and may, if they have the opportunity, lay them in wounds or sores on the skin of man. The maggots then live in the pus and other material that they find in these sores. Thus flesh flies belonging to the genus *Sarcophaga*, which are common in Europe, America, Asia, and Africa and lay, not eggs, but larvae that have hatched out inside the fly, may lay these larvae in wounds and sores on human skin; and their relatives belonging to the genus *Wohlfahrtia*, which occurs in southern

Europe (but not in Britain), Asia, and Africa, have the same habit. The females of some species of this genus will attack healthy human skin.

Related to the species just mentioned, but belonging to the group of calliphorine flies to which the bluebottle flies belong, are species which do not usually attack healthy skin, but will attack it when there is no more than a flea bite or some other small wound. They are also attracted by the odours coming from such organs as the nose or mouth or eye or vagina when these organs are diseased; but the danger of these species is that their larvae feed on living flesh and may cause horrible deformations that often end in death. Their maggots are called screw-worms and there are three important species of these screw-worm flies. *Callitroga hominivorax* (= *C. americana*), the American screw-worm fly, occurs in the Americas from the southern United States as far south as northern Chile and southern Brazil. *Chrysomyia bezziana*, the maggots of which may cause horrible lesions, is found in Africa, India, and other parts of southern Asia. *Callitroga macellaria* is found in Canada, the United States, and South America; usually this fly breeds in dead carcasses and only invades wounds after bacteria have developed in them and have made them foul. *Chrysomyia megacephala* is a species that also lays eggs in foul wounds, but occurs in the Old World.

Two other species of calliphorine flies may attack man in tropical Africa. These are *Cordylobia anthropophaga*, the tumbu fly, a yellowish-brown fly which lays its eggs in dry sand or clothing left exposed to flies. The larvae that emerge bore, when they get the opportunity, into the skins of rodents, which they prefer, or into the skin of man and other animals, and bury themselves there, causing the formation of small tumours resembling boils, in which the larvae become mature in about eight days. They then leave the skin to pupate on the ground.

Another species, *Auchmeromyia luteola*, the larva of which is the well-known Congo floor maggot, is also a pest of man in tropical Africa. It is parasitic on man alone and is, according to Chandler (1955), the only fly that is. The yellowish-brown adult flies are not parasitic. They feed on human excreta and decaying vegetable material near human dwellings and lay their eggs in the dust along the edges of the mats on which the natives sleep on the earthern floor. The eggs hatch in about two days and the larvae feed, usually at night, by puncturing the skin of man and sucking blood. During the day they lie hidden in the dust under the mats. The life history occupies about ten weeks. The bites do not usually cause serious irritation.

THE WARBLE FLIES AND THEIR RELATIVES

The habits of such species as the tumbu fly recall those of the warble flies and their relatives, which belong to the group of insects called the Oestridae, the larvae of which are parasitic in the skin or the internal organs of man and other animals. The adult flies, which are not parasitic, have short antennae partly sunk in grooves on the sides of the head and they cannot feed because their mouth parts are degenerate. Their larvae are covered with spines arranged in various ways. Some species of them, such as the warble flies of cattle and the bot flies of horses, lay eggs which they attach to the hairs of these hosts; others, such as the sheep nasal fly and the sheep ked, lay, not eggs, but larvae which have developed in the female insect's womb.

The larvae of the warble flies of cattle, when they emerge from the eggs attached in the summer to the hairs of the cattle, penetrate the skin of the host and live through the succeeding winter inside the bodies of the cattle. First they wander to the walls of the gullet and later to the tissues of the back on either side of the spine. Here they mature, causing as they do so, the formation of swellings, called warbles, which are really abscesses, on the pus of which the larvae feed. Each larva cuts a small hole in the skin through which it breathes and these holes reduce the value of the leather and cause considerable losses to the leather trade. The meat is also damaged, so that the meat trade also suffers.

When they are mature, the larvae drop to the ground and

pupate there. Occasionally the warble flies of cattle lay their eggs on other hosts. Horses, for example, may be attacked and several instances are known of the occurrence of the larvae of the warble flies of cattle in the skin of man, especially in the skin of people living on farms. These larvae do not, however, usually reach maturity in these unusual hosts, though they may cause annoying sores in man. In race horses they may affect the saddle-area and prevent the horses from racing.

In South America, however, from northern Argentina up to Mexico, man is also attacked by a warble fly, *Dermatobia hominis*, which also attacks cattle and causes farmers considerable loss. This fly, which is rather bigger than a bluebottle fly and has a predominantly bluish or violet colour, has a remarkable method of getting its eggs to the hosts on which its larvae are parasitic. It does not attach them to the hairs of these hosts. It sends them instead hitch-hiking on the abdomen of another insect. The insects most often chosen are the large and beautiful mosquitoes belonging to the genus *Psorophora*. The female *Dermatobia* captures one of these, or she may capture other two-winged blood-sucking flies or even ticks, and glues her eggs to the abdomen of the captured insect or tick. These blood-suckers then fly to feed on a warm-blooded vertebrate host and the larvae of *Dermatobia* emerge and penetrate the skin of the warm-blooded animal. The blood-sucking habit of the transport host is thus used as a means of getting the eggs to the host in which they can develop.

Inside the egg of *Dermatobia hominis* a larva develops which leaves the egg and penetrates into the skin of the warm-blooded host. These larvae (fig. 61) develop further and they are, at a later stage of their development, covered, as the larvae of the warble flies of cattle also are, with spines, which irritate the tissues of the host. They cause, as the larvae of the ox warble flies also do, a reaction of the host which encloses the larvae in a fibrous bag or cyst. Opening into this cyst is a small hole to which the larva applies its hinder end where its spiracles are, so that it can breathe air. The larvae, when they are mature, drop out of the skin of the host and turn into pupae on the ground. The whole life history requires three or four months, so that it is considerably shorter than that of the warble flies of cattle.

The cysts in which the larvae develop occur most often on exposed parts of the human body, such as the hands, wrists, ankles, neck, and face; but they may occur elsewhere. Craig and Faust (1955) record that the eggs may be laid on damp laundry hung out to dry and that the larvae may then enter the

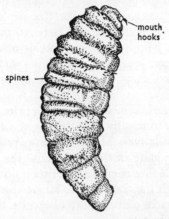

Fig. 61. Full-grown larva of the human
warble fly, *Dermatobia hominis*

skin when the clothes are later put on. The cysts are very painful and they may itch unbearably. Even after the larvae have been killed by nicotine in tobacco juice applied to the cysts, or better, by the newer insecticides, such as Lindane, or by plugging the breathing holes of the larvae with fat, or by other methods, such as surgical removal of the grubs, the wounds left may, if they are not kept clean and aseptic, become infected with bacteria, or with the screw-worms mentioned above, and serious lesions may then be caused.

The fact that the larvae of flies of the genus *Hypoderma*, which cause warbles of cattle, may occasionally develop to a certain extent, although they cannot mature, in the skin of man, is paralleled by the fact that the larvae of the sheep nasal fly, *Oestrus ovis*, which produces, not eggs, but larvae,

239

may develop in the nasal passages of man if the flies lay them there. Normally this fly lays her larvae in the nasal passages of sheep, but man may also be attacked in this way, shepherds being especially liable to attack. In the nasal passages of sheep these spined larvae, which have powerful mouth-hooks, develop during the winter in the recesses of the nose and may cause severe inflammation there. They may travel up the nose into the sinuses in the bones behind the nose, or even into the brain. A related species, called the Russian gadfly, attacks horses and cattle in southern and eastern Europe, northern Africa, and Asia Minor and this species also may attack man. Other related species of these flies attack camels in north Africa, and Asia and deer in Europe and North America.

The larvae of the horse bot flies, which belong to the genus *Gasterophilus*, are normally parasitic in the food canals of horses and their relatives. The adult non-parasitic flies attach their eggs to the hairs of their hosts and the larvae, unlike those of the warble flies of cattle, enter their hosts through the mouth, or through the cheeks. The larvae then attach themselves to the stomachs of the hosts and develop there until they become mature. They are then passed out of the host in its excreta and they become pupae on the ground outside the host. Occasionally the larvae of one species of these flies, *Gasterophilus intestinalis*, may enter the skin of man and wander about under the skin, causing a condition called *larva migrans* or wandering larva. This name is, however, usually given, as was explained in chapter 3, to infection of the skin with the larvae of the strains of the nematode hookworm of the dog and cat, *Ancylostoma braziliense*.

To the 'itches' caused by larvae of parasitic animals that penetrate into human skin can be added those caused by the cercariae of flukes. The skin-penetrating cercariae, for instance, of the blood-flukes described in chapter 5, and those of related species, cause an itching inflammation of the skin when they enter the skin of man and wander about in it. This kind of inflammation may be caused by the cercariae of flukes the adult stages of which cannot be parasitic in man. Thus the name 'swamp-itch' is given to inflammation of the skin caused by the cercariae of *Schistosoma spindalis* (*S. spindale*), the adults of which are parasitic in sheep and cattle in India, Malaya, and South Africa; and the cercariae of flukes the adults of which are parasitic in birds, such as ducks, or in other vertebrates, such as mice, may get into the skins of people bathing from the shores of the Great Lakes of Canada and the northern United States, or in New Zealand, India, France, Germany, and Wales. These cercariae come from snails of the genera *Physa* and *Limnaea*, which are the intermediate hosts of these flukes and they cause an itching inflammation of the skin called *swimmer's itch*. A similar inflammation called *collector's itch* may affect naturalists collecting specimens from muddy or swampy areas in Michigan, which are inhabited by snails that are the intermediate hosts of unidentified flukes the adults of which cannot live in man. All these forms of inflammation of the skin are to be regarded as successful, but annoying, reactions of man to a parasite which cannot attain maturity in his body.

ARACHNIDA

The general features of the Class Arachnida have been given briefly in chapter 2 and their mouth parts have been described earlier in this chapter. Here we are concerned only with the ticks and mites, which belong to the Order Acarina. The bodies of species of this Order are usually somewhat globular and they usually do not show external division into segments. Their mouth parts (fig. 54) have been described above. The ticks are, as a rule, larger than the mites, most of which are small, or even minute. All ticks (Ixodoidea) are parasitic, but all mites are not. Among the mites are many species which live non-parasitic lives either in the water or on land, some of the latter being serious pests of grain, flour, and other stored products. Sometimes these latter get on to the skins of people who handle these products and cause inflammations of the skin known as baker's itch, grocer's itch, and other similar names.

Ticks

Ticks are divided into soft ticks (Argasidae) and hard ticks (Ixodidae). These names refer to the fact that the bodies of soft ticks (fig. 62) are leathery, soft, and often covered with small projections called mammillae, while the bodies of hard ticks (fig. 63 and Plate 7) are covered with a firmer chitinous covering, on the dorsal side of which, on the back of the tick, there is a chitinous plate called the *scutum* (fig. 63). The male hard tick is smaller than the female hard tick and often does not suck blood; its scutum is much larger than that of the

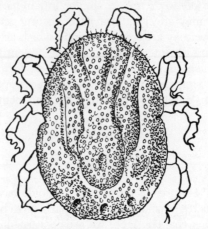

Fig. 62. A soft tick (*Ornithodoros mou-bata*), showing the mammillae on the surface

blood-sucking female. The bodies of some species of hard ticks have patches of enamel-like colour and there may be ventral thickenings of the integument called plates or shields. At the hind end there may be grooves marking out areas called *festoons* (fig. 64). Soft ticks have no scutum and none of them have plates or shields. The mouth parts of soft ticks are, moreover, hidden in a groove called the *camerostome* below the anterior end of the body, so that they cannot be seen from above; the mouthparts and capitulum of hard ticks (fig. 54), on the

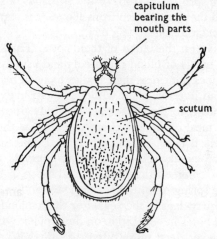

Fig. 63. A hard tick (*Ixodes ricinus*). Male, showing the large scutum and the mouthparts

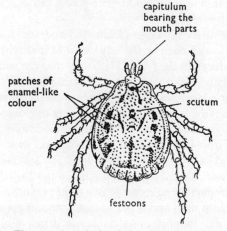

Fig. 64. A male hard tick (*Dermacentor variabilis*), showing the festoons and the enamel-like patches of colour that some species of hard ticks, called ornate ticks, have

other hand, project in front of the tick and look rather like a small head that can be seen from above. It is sometimes called the *rostrum* or false head (fig 63).

Ticks live on the blood of their hosts. The soft ticks take moderate meals of blood repeatedly and usually at night and the meal does not cause their bodies to swell markedly. Some of them can live for years without blood; individuals of one species known to the writer have already lived fifteen years without a meal of blood and are still alive as these words are written. Hard ticks, on the other hand, take large meals of blood, but they take these only at long intervals. Some species, such as the common tick of cattle and sheep in England, feed only in the spring or autumn of each year and only for a period of about thirty days in the year. For the remainder of the year the female hides in vegetation on the ground. Other species of ticks, however, feed more often than this. When these relatively large meals are taken, the body of the female hard tick swells up markedly, the fully-fed tick being called an *engorged tick*, while the unfed tick is called a *flat tick*. The males of hard ticks do not often feed on blood. The young of ticks, however, feed much as the adults do.

The female ticks lay eggs (Plate 7b) and some species of them carefully wax each of the eggs as it is laid with a waxy secretion produced in the head. Then they toss the waxed eggs over on to their backs and may be almost buried by them. From the egg a larva, called the *seed-tick*, emerges, which has only three pairs of legs, as an insect has. It can, however, be distinguished from an insect by its lack of antennae and segmentation of the body and by its possession of chelicerae, pedipalps, and a hypostome. The larva is succeeded by a nymph with four pairs of legs and then becomes the adult tick.

Ticks are important to man for two chief reasons. They remove blood from man and other animals, and, if they are numerous, they may remove appreciable quantities of blood; but this is less important than the irritation that their bites cause. The wounds produced by the bites may also become infected by bacteria, so that sores result, or they may attract the flies mentioned above which lay their eggs or larvae in wounds on the surface of the skin. Injury inflicted in these ways is, however, much less important than the injury ticks do by transmitting the causes of serious and often fatal diseases to man and other animals. Not only do they transmit to domesticated animals such serious diseases as redwater fever (babesiasis) and East Coast fever (theileriasis), and similar diseases of sheep and horses, which may cause severe losses of these valuable animals, but they also transmit to man a number of diseases that are among the most serious afflictions of man. It is impossible here to describe them all, or to discuss at length the complex details of the manner in which ticks transmit them, but a few examples of them can be given.

Many species of the genus of soft ticks, *Ornithodoros*, transmit to man and other animals the spirochaetes which cause relapsing fever in tropical and north Africa, western Asia, Central and South America, the western United States and Canada, and Spain. *Ornithodoros moubata* (fig. 62), which is mainly a parasite of man and lives in human dwellings, transmits this disease in tropical Africa. *O. savignyi*, which does not normally inhabit human dwellings, transmits it in Africa and western Asia. In northern South America the species concerned is *O. rudis* and in California *O. hermsi*.

Ticks also transmit to man and other animals diseases caused by the organisms belonging to the genus *Rickettsia*, which are not bacteria or viruses, but are, in many respects, intermediate between these. Ticks, for instance, transmit to man North American or Rocky Mountain Spotted Fever, caused by *Rickettsia rickettsii*. This disease occurs in the western United States and Canada, and similar diseases, caused by other species of the genus *Rickettsia*, occur in countries bordering the Mediterranean sea, in tropical and South Africa, India and adjacent regions, and northern Australia. The ticks which transmit these diseases to man and other animals belong to the genera *Dermacentor* (fig. 64), *Amblyomma*, *Rhipicephalus*, *Haemaphysalis*, and perhaps other genera.

Another disease of man and other animals caused by a *Rickettsia* (*Coxiella*) *burneti* is *Q fever*. It occurs in the United States, Australia, where it was discovered in 1937, the Medi-

terranean area, Africa, and Switzerland. The disease resembles influenza in some respects, and ticks are suspected of
being vectors of it; but the evidence in favour of this is not
conclusive and the disease is frequently acquired without the
intervention of any vector.

Tularaemia, a disease of rabbits and other rodents caused by
a bacillus called *Pasteurella tularensis,* which is related to the
bacillus that causes plague, may cause a serious disease of man.
It is transmitted to man by species of the genera *Dermacentor,*
possibly by *Amblyomma americanum* and also by blood-sucking
tabanid and deerflies and by fleas, lice, bed-bugs, and contact
with persons suffering from the disease. Among other diseases transmitted by ticks are some that are caused by filterable
viruses, such as American mountain fever (Colorado tick
fever) transmitted by *Dermacentor andersoni* and Russian
Spring-Summer encephalitis, which the tick *Ixodes persulcatus*
transmits to man in European Russia, Siberia, and far-eastern
Russia in the Spring and Summer. *Dermacentor andersoni* may
transmit to man a form of human encephalitis in the western
United States and also an encephalitis of horses. A form of
paralysis called tick-paralysis, which is accompanied by fever
and other symptoms and may end in death, is communicated
to sheep and cattle and dogs by *Dermacentor andersoni* and
other species of this genus in North America and Canada and
it may infect man, especially children.

Mites

Apart from the ticks, man and other animals are annoyed by
many smaller parasitic species related to the ticks, which are
often lumped together as mites. There is a great variety of
these species and all the species that annoy man, or communicate diseases to him, cannot be described in this book. Species
that injure crops, such as the gall mites or blister mites that attack certain fruits, grapes, peaches, plums, and also onions,
garlic, and other plants and others that damage stored products, such as grain and flour and may get on to human skin
and cause an annoying dermatitis, have been mentioned above.

A species that may annoy man directly especially during the

late summer and autumn is *Trombicula autumnalis,* the larvae of which are called 'harvesters', or berry bugs or bracken bugs or, in Ireland, orange-tawneys. They should not be confused with the harvest-men, which are bigger adult arachnids belonging to the Order Phalangidea. These minute, reddish larvae, which are only about 0·2 to 0·5 mm. long and about half as broad, suck the lymph and blood from man and other mammals, causing the formation, at the sites of their bites, of papules which itch intensely and are often called 'heat-spots'. Dogs may be considerably annoyed by these larvae, which attack them between the toes. The larvae puncture the skin and inject into it a substance that dissolves the skin and forms a kind of tube through which the larva feeds. When it is mature the larva becomes a nymph, which later becomes the adult mite, but neither the nymph nor the adult sucks blood. The larvae are often abundant in late summer and autumn on grass or heathland, especially on sandy soils. Relatives of them, the larvae of *Trombicula akamushi* and perhaps those of other species of this genus also, transmit to man the Rickettsial organism that causes the disease called mite-typhus, scrub-typhus, tsutsu-gamushi disease, or Japanese river fever, which attacked the Allied troops severely during the Second World War.

Another species that may transmit serious disease to man is the gamasid mite, *Ornithonyssus* (*Liponyssus*) *bacoti,* which is called the tropical rat mite. It transmits, from rats to man and man to man, the Rickettsial organism that causes endemic (murine) typhus and possibly also the Rickettsias that cause Q fever and other diseases.

Belonging to a different family is *Demodex folliculorum* (fig. 65), the mite that lives in the pits out of which the hairs of dogs and other mammals grow and causes the disease called follicular or demodectic mange. The bodies of these mites are elongated in adaptation to their lives in the narrow hair-follicles, an adaptation which recalls that of some species of feather-mites, which live inside the quills of the feathers of the fowl and other birds. There are several varieties of the species *Demodex folliculorum,* each of which has a different host. Thus one variety, attacks man, another the dog, another the sheep, and others attack the goat, the ox, and other animals. The variety that may be found in the hair-follicles of man, or in the sebaceous glands that secrete a lubricant substance and open into these follicles, does not usually cause a serious disease and often it causes no disease at all. It has been suggested that it causes the formation of 'blackheads' on the skin of man, but

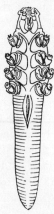

Fig. 65. A mite (*Demodex folliculorum*),
the cause of demodectic mange

there is doubt about this. In dogs, this species causes the serious disease called demodectic mange, which may take either the form called scaly or red mange, in which the reddened or coppery, scaly, and wrinkled skin itches intensely, or the pustular form, in which infection with bacteria occurs and abscesses form. In either form the dogs acquire a repulsive smell and suffer intensely. The disease is eradicated only with great difficulty.

The remaining mites which attack man belong to the group called the Sarcoptiformes, which includes the remarkable, harmless, and often very beautiful oribatid mites which live on pastures, under moss and in similar places, and the mites which belong to the families Psoroptidae and Sarcoptidae. The family Psoroptidae includes species which do not burrow in the skin of the host. Among them are (1) species of the genus

Psoroptes, which cause psoroptic mange of sheep (sheep-scab), a horrible disease that is now rapidly being eradicated from all progressive farms by means of the newer acaricides and the vigilance of veterinarians and farmers, and psoroptic mange of horses, cattle, sheep, and goats; (2) species of the genus *Otodectes*, which attack the canal leading to the ear drums of dogs, cats, and their relatives; and (3) species of the genus *Chorioptes*, which cause chorioptic mange of the feet of horses. The family Sarcoptidae includes species which do burrow into the substance of the skin. It includes (1) species of the genus *Sarcoptes*, which attack man causing scabies; and varieties of this species which cause sarcoptic mange of horses, cattle, sheep, pigs, and other animals; (2) species of the genus *Notoedres*, which causes a similar disease of the face and ears of cats and rabbits; and (3) species of the genus *Cnemidocoptes*, which cause the disease called scaly-leg of poultry, parrots, and other birds, and depluming itch, which causes the feathers of poultry and other birds to fall out. We are concerned in this book chiefly with the species of the genus *Sarcoptes* and especially with a variety of the species *Sarcoptes scabiei*, which attacks man and causes scabies. It should be remembered, however, that sarcoptic mange of the other animals mentioned above is caused by varieties of this species, many of which, although they each normally attack only the animals to which they are adapted, will, if circumstances are favourable, attack the skin of man and live in it for a time. The varieties of *Sarcoptes scabiei* that cause sarcoptic mange of horses and pigs are perhaps especially liable to establish themselves temporarily in the skin of man and to cause an annoying dermatitis that may require treatment.

The human variety of *Sarcoptes scabiei* (Plate 8) is a small, somewhat globular, semi-transparent mite, the largest phase of which, the egg-laying female, measures about 0·3 by 0·26 mm. (about $\frac{1}{100}$ inch), the males measuring 0·2 by 0·16 mm. Their detailed structure need not concern us here, except to mention the interesting fact that the mites, in all their phases, have, on some of their four pairs of legs, peculiar stalked suckers with which they walk. The suckers have been aptly compared by

Mellanby (1943) to bell-shaped flaps of washleather and the mites adhere by means of them to surfaces over which they walk. Inside the egg-laying (*ovigerous*) females the ovoid, transparent egg in its thin shell can be seen. Usually only one or two eggs can be seen in the body at a time. The egg looks enormous, because it measures 0·15 by 0·1 mm., which is about a third of the size of the mite's body. The eggs are laid in burrows excavated in human skin by the egg-laying female mite. She leaves them behind her in a row, attached to the floor of the burrow as she moves along at the rate of about 0·5 to 5 mm. a day. She burrows with her chelicerae and also uses cutting plates on the last segment of the first two pairs of legs, so that she looks, as Mellanby (1943) said, as if she was digging with her mouth parts and elbows.

The eggs hatch in three to five days and liberate a larva, which is like the adults in general, but has only three pairs of legs. The larvae either stay in the burrow in which they hatch, or make new burrows out of this at an angle to it. They feed and grow for four to six days and then moult the skin to become the nymph, which has, like the adult, four pairs of legs. The nymphs excavate their own burrows and moult in about two days to become either adult males, or what are called *pubescent*, that is to say, unfertilized, *females*. The males usually make short burrows of their own, in which they stay for a short time before they leave them to spend most of their lives on the surface of the skin, where they search for the females. The pubescent females also make their own burrows and, when they are fertilized, they become the egg-laying or *ovigerous* females.

Many of these various phases of the mites die or are killed in or on the skin and Mellanby (1943) found that, among 900 people suffering from scabies, the average number of adult female mites per person was only 11·3 and that the females are chiefly responsible for the symptoms of this disease. More than half of these 900 people had only 1 to 5 mites. It must be remembered, however, that the number of the other phases of the life history present was probably more than 20 times that of the adult females. These small numbers of mites are in great contrast to the thousands of the other species of mites mentioned above that may be present on domesticated and other animals.

The mites cause inflammation of the human skin and the well-known itching characteristic of the disease. The hands and wrists are most often affected, but other parts of the body may be attacked. The first signs of the disease are reddening of the skin and rings of papules several inches wide appear and then the itching begins. It causes the sufferer to scratch and scratching may aggravate the inflammation and it may liberate fluid from vesicles underneath the burrows made by the mites. This fluid dries and scabs form and bacteria may be introduced, so that septic sores may result. The itching may not begin for a month or longer after the infection is acquired. It cannot, therefore, be due to the movements of the mites. Mellanby (1943) considers that it is due to sensitization of the infected person. Infection is probably conveyed directly from one person to another, but experts disagree as to whether the female mites or the larvae and nymphs are chiefly responsible for transmitting it.

Pentastomids

One other Order of the Arachnida remains to be briefly considered. This is the Order Pentastomida, which includes the organisms called tongueworms, linguatulids, or pentastomes. These are parasitic arachnids with indirect life histories, which have been so much altered by parasitic life that their bodies (fig. 66) look more like the bodies of worms than arthropods. The adults are parasitic in reptiles, birds, and mammals. They are usually elongated animals with a skin marked externally by transverse striations or deep rings, which help to give these animals their worm-like appearance; but they have, at the anterior end, two pairs of hooked claws which are degenerate arthropod limbs and their whole structure and development shows that they are arthropods. The sexes are separate and the eggs, when they are laid, contain a fully-developed larva, which hatches out and is swallowed by an intermediate host, inside which the nymph is parasitic, usually inside a cyst. The nymph infects the final host.

Animals Parasitic in Man

Linguatulids are important because the larvae and nymphs of some species have been found in the liver, spleen and lungs of man in Africa in Egypt, Gambia, Senegal, the Ivory and Gold Coasts, and in the Belgian Congo. These belong to the species *Armillifer armillatus*. Immature stages of *Armillifer moniliformis* have also been found in man in China, Manila and Java. Certain snakes are the normal intermediate hosts of

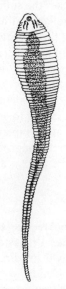

Fig. 66. The tongueworm of the dog,
Linguatula serrata

these species and man probably acquired them by eating these snakes. The nymphs of the tongue worm of the dog, *Linguatula serrata* (fig. 66), which inhabits the nose and neighbouring passages of dogs and perhaps other carnivorous mamals, have also been found in man in Africa, the Panama Canal area, Brazil, Switzerland, and Germany; and in one human being only, a patient examined in Texas, the adult of this species has been found. There have also been reports of the occurrence of *Armillifer armillatus* in the nose of man.

Usually the nymphs cause no symptoms in man, but rarely

they may cause congestion of the lungs or abdominal pain and jaundice or even intestinal obstruction. In sheep and cattle the nymphs of the tongueworm of the dog may be numerous and it may be difficult to distinguish the lesions they cause from those of tuberculosis.

CHAPTER ELEVEN

Gain and Loss for the Parasite

━━━━━━

IT has often been said that parasitic animals are degenerate. This statement, true though it may be of some species not parasitic in man, is certainly not true of all the species of parasitic animals. There are some which have lost, as a result of a long history of parasitic life, so much of the structure of their ancestors that biologists can trace their ancestry only by studying the development of the individual, which so frequently indicates the origins of all kinds of animals, whether they are parasitic or not. The crustacean parasite, *Sacculina*, for instance, which is related to the barnacles, is, in its adult state, little more than a sac containing sexual organs, which is attached to the abdomen of the crab which is its host and it feeds by means of tubes which ramify inside the crab's body. The crustacean ancestry of this species was proved by the discovery that its development includes a larval stage of the type called a *nauplius larva*, which is characteristic of the Crustacea. Among the species described in this book the degenerate pentastomid arthropods described in chapter 10 also show loss of much of the structure characteristic of their relatives; they look like worms, but are in reality related to the king-crabs, scorpion and spiders. But species like these are examples of the more extreme degrees of structural alteration caused by parasitic life. Such species are degenerate only in the sense that they have lost some, or it may be almost all, of the organs that their non-parasitic relatives have. In other respects they are, not degenerate, but highly specialized for their particular mode of life. Physiologically they may be very remarkably adapted to this mode of life. When, in fact, we review the whole range of parasitic animals, we can hardly deny that they show both structural and physiological adaptations that are not only very efficient, but beautiful as well. If we add to this the remarkable correlation that we find between the life histories of parasitic animals and the life histories of their hosts, the idea that parasitic animals are degenerate becomes quite untenable. They are, on the contrary, among the most specialized of living things and the preceding pages, which describe only the animals parasitic on man, will have left no doubt of the success in life that parasitic animals achieve. To support this argument further, let us look, in this chapter, at some of the structural and physiological changes that the species described in earlier chapters have undergone.

For brevity and clarity these changes will be classified as changes caused by the method of feeding, changes caused by the need to hold on to the host, changes due to reduction or loss of particular organs that are not needed for parasitic life, modifications of the reproductive processes, and correlation between the life histories of the parasitic animals and the life histories of their hosts, some of which have been indicated in the earlier chapters of this book. This classification of these changes does not include the interesting and remarkable modifications of respiratory and some other physiological processes, that some species of parasitic animals show, but we shall not have space to describe these and must be content with the indications of them given in earlier chapters.

CHANGES DUE TO THE METHOD OF FEEDING AND ATTACHMENT TO THE HOST

These two types of structural modifications of parasitic animals can be considered together because they are very often correlated with one another. The most important of the methods by which animals parasitic in man obtain their food have been indicated in the account of these species given above. Naturally they affect, in many species, the region of the mouth. The hookworms, for instance, develop efficient teeth and the whole structure of the mouth-region proclaims their habit of browsing on the lining of the small intestine of the host and penetrating below this lining to suck blood. The sucking is performed by a muscular pharynx behind the mouth and many other species of parasitic animals develop a sucking pharynx of this type. The leeches parasitic on man also possess small denticles on their jaws, although their relatives, belonging to another group of leeches, the Rhynchobdellidae, which include species which suck the blood of fishes and transmit trypanosomes to the fish, feed by means of a muscular proboscis which can be everted for feeding or withdrawn into the body. The blood-sucking bat, *Desmodus*, has enlarged incisor teeth with sharp edges, which enable it to scoop out pieces of the flesh of its victims. The hag-fishes also have teeth on their powerful tongues and one tooth on the roof of the mouth. More complex are the modifications of the mouth parts of insects, ticks, and mites that suck the blood or other tissue fluids of their hosts. These modifications are described in chapter 10.

A different method of feeding is employed by the roundworms belonging to the genus *Trichuris* (Plate 2b). Worms of this type are called whipworms, because the anterior twothirds or so of the body is thin and threadlike, while the posterior third is thicker, so that the whole worm looks rather like a whip, with its lash attached.

Whipworms feed by thrusting the thin anterior end into the lining of the caecum or colon of the host and injecting into this a digestive fluid which converts the tissues around the mouth into a liquid which the worm sucks up. These worms therefore make for themselves a soup which they imbibe. The long, thin anterior end of the worm serves at the same time to attach the worm to its host. This is a good example of the combination in one organ of the functions of feeding and attachment to the host. The mouth parts of blood-sucking insects perform the same two functions, although they are less efficient for holding on to the host. The toothed hypostome of the ticks, on the other hand, which has recurved teeth, which prevent withdrawal of the blood-sucking mouth parts, is a very effective means of holding on to the host.

The hooks and suckers of the tapeworms and flukes seem, at first sight, to be less efficient than some other methods of attachment to the host, but this is true only of the species of these animals that are parasitic in man. A glance at the formidable clamps and hooks of flukes and tapeworms which use hosts other than man leaves us in no doubt about their efficiency as organs of attachment, and, even among the species parasitic in man, the muscular suckers and hooks are astonishingly effective. This is especially true of such relatively bulky and weighty species as the beef and fish tapeworms, although these are no doubt helped by being buoyed up in the fluid contents of the host's food canal. The hooklets of the hexacanth embryos of tapeworms have the different function of enabling these embryos to tear their way through the tissues of the host after they have entered into the body. Consideration of the tapeworms reminds us of the manner in which these remarkable creatures feed. Unlike the flukes, they have lost all traces of the mouth and food canal. They feed by absorbing certain elements of the host's food through their soft skins, a habit that can succeed only when the parasitic animal lives in a nutritive fluid inside the body of the host. Such species as the trypanosomes and other species that live in the blood and lymph, feed on these fluids, which are, as the blood-sucking species have found out, rich sources of essential food materials.

Among other organs developed by the adult phases of parasitic animals for holding on to the host are the claws on the feet of such parasitic insects as the fleas and lice and the peculiar suckers on some of the legs of mites. Nor must we forget the methods by which the adults of some species attach their eggs to the host. Species described in this book which do this are the lice, warble flies, and horse bot flies which attach their eggs to the host's hairs.

REDUCTION OR LOSS OF ORGANS

Many parasitic animals, once they have established themselves inside the body of a host, tend to lead inactive lives. They find their food supply, live on it, and reproduce their kind and then the adults die. It might be expected, therefore, that a relatively inactive life of this kind, which causes, among nonparasitic animals, reduction or loss of organs, would also cause reduction or loss of organs by parasitic animals. It does seem to do this. Inactive life, however, and the consequences that it involves, are characteristic mainly of the adult phases of parasitic animals. Their larval phases, and especially the infective larval phases that have to make contact with a host, are frequently active creatures which lead lives that are not very different from those of animals that are not parasitic. For this reason any reductions or losses of organs that we find among parasitic animals are more characteristic of the adult phases.

So far as digestive organs are concerned, the tapeworms alone, among the species described in this book, show complete absence of the food canal and its accessory glands. The thorny-headed worms (Acanthocephala), which are only occasionally parasitic in man, also have no food canal. Among the other parasitic worms described in this book, the flukes have by no means lost the food canal; it is, among them, a branched tube, which may have secondary, and even tertiary, branches. Among the roundworms the food canal is a straight and largely undifferentiated tube, but a prominent feature of it is the muscular pharynx which sucks the food in. A muscular pharyngeal pump is also found among the parasitic insects and arachnids that suck blood.

The loss or reduction of locomotor organs is a more conspicuous feature of parasitic life. The adult phases of roundworms, tapeworms, and flukes have no special locomotor organs, but the absence of these among these species can hardly be regarded as a consequence of parasitic life, because these worms belong to a stage in the evolution of animals at which the development of paired limbs, at any rate, had not yet been accomplished. It is among the parasitic arthropods that we find the most conspicuous examples of the modification or loss of locomotor organs. The presence of only one pair of wings in parasitic dipterous insects such as the tsetse flies and the horse flies is not an example of loss of organs due to parasitic life, because all the Diptera have only one pair of wings and most of them are not parasitic. The complete loss of wings by such insects as the lice and fleas, correlated as it is with the development of claws on the feet and the flattening of

Gain and Loss for the Parasite

the bodies of lice and the lateral compression of the bodies of fleas, is, however, undoubtedly associated with their parasitic life on the surfaces of their hosts bodies. We can, in fact, trace, among the members of the family of dipterous insects called the Hippoboscidae, all stages between parasitic species such as the forest fly, *Hippobosca equina*, found on horses in the New Forest and elsewhere, which has clawed feet with adhesive pads but has retained its wings, through species the females of which keep their wings till they reach the host and then cast them off, to such wingless species as the sheep-ked, which lives, much as a louse does, in the wool of sheep.

Among other parasitic arthropods there are many examples of the loss of the locomotor organs that their near relatives possess, but few of these are parasitic in man, so that they are not described in this book. An account of them is given by Lapage (1951) and by other authors mentioned in the bibliography at the end of this book. The pentastomid species described in chapter 10 do, however, show reduction of the limbs to mere stumps provided with hooks, and the mite, *Demodex folliculorum*, described in the same chapter, also has limbs reduced in size and number.

The reduction in size or number of locomotor organs, or even the complete loss of them, does not necessarily mean that the parasitic animal cannot move about. It may be correlated with an efficient muscular system that enables the parasitic animal to lead a remarkably active life. The parasitic maggots of such insects as the blowflies are, for example, very active and anyone who has seen the maggot of a sheep nasal fly wriggling away from capture in the nasal passages of a sheep will have no doubt of the speed and agility of these legless pests.

Nor should we forget that, although parasitic life does cause reduction or loss of locomotor organs by some species of parasitic animals, it also causes the development by other species of new structures that are improvements from the parasite's point of view. The trypanosomes, for example, which live in the blood of their hosts, which is a relatively viscid medium, develop the undulating membrane described in chapter 9 and species of the genus *Trichomonas*, which live in the mucoid secretion of the human vagina, have developed a similar organ, which helps them to move in fluids of this nature. The peculiar and very efficient bell-shaped suckers on some or all of the legs of the mites described in chapter 10 are also examples of the development of new organs that are specialized for locomotory purposes.

Modifications of Reproductive Processes

The animals parasitic in man do not show us all the remarkable modifications of reproductive processes that are associated with parasitic life, but they do introduce us to some of the most important of them. They have been indicated in the preceding chapters, but a brief account of them here will emphasize the fact that parasitic life entails a high mortality – and in some species an enormous mortality – among the young of the parasitic animal. This is true especially of the species whose eggs or larvae must leave the host and lead for a time a non-parasitic life, at the end of which they have the problem of making contact with a host. Failure to make successful contact with a host means death for the infective phase whose task it is, and, if the majority of the infective phases fail to make contact with the host, the species itself to which they belong may fail to survive. Life inside the host also has its difficulties, because the host reacts against the parasite. It is not surprising, therefore, that parasitic animals have evolved methods of dealing with factors both inside and outside the host that may threaten the survival of the species to which they belong. These adaptations can be summed up as adaptations which increase the numbers of eggs and sperms produced, those that facilitate the fertilization of the eggs and those that increase the number of individuals derived from each egg.

(1) *Increase in the number of eggs or sperms produced* may be effected by increase in the size or number of the ovaries and testes that produce them or increase in the capacity of a relatively small ovary to produce eggs. Both are well shown by the parasitic flukes and tapeworms.

The hermaphrodite sexual organs of the flukes occupy the greater part of the fluke's body. Those of tapeworms are serially repeated in each of the segments of the body of the tapeworm. In some species, indeed, such as the dog tapeworm, *Dipylidium caninum*, mentioned in chapter 6, there may be two sets of them in each of these segments. Because tapeworms develop a large number of these segments, the number of fertilized eggs produced may be enormous. The fish tapeworm, *Diphyllobothrium latum*, for example, may produce 36,000 to a million eggs a day. Each of the gravid segments of the beef tapeworm, *Taenia saginata*, may, although the ovary in it is comparatively small, contain an average of 97,000 eggs; there may be 1,000 to 2,000 gravid segments and the average number of eggs produced each year by this species has been estimated to be 594 million. This tapeworm can live in man for ten years and it is not to be supposed that it can go on producing eggs at this rate throughout its life, but the number of eggs it produces during its lifetime is certainly remarkable. The pork tapeworm, *Taenia solium*, does not produce so many eggs. Each gravid segment contains only 30,000 to 50,000 eggs and it does not usually have more than 1,000 segments.

Large numbers of eggs are also produced by some of the roundworms, in which the ovary is a long, coiled structure, which is relatively larger than the ovaries of flukes and tapeworms. One of the star performers in this group of worms is the large roundworm of man, *Ascaris lumbricoides*, a single female of which may contain, at any one time, about 27 million eggs, about 200,000 of which are laid each day. A reasonable estimate of the annual output of fertilized eggs is therefore 60 to 70 million and some 75 per cent of these remain for many months, and, under favourable circumstances, for as long as five years, capable of infecting new hosts. The human hookworm, *Ancylostoma duodenale*, produces some 25,000 to 35,000 eggs a day and may lay, during its lifetime of five years or so, a total of 18 to 54 million eggs. The other important species of human hookworms, *Necator americanus*, produces fewer eggs. Its females lay about 6,000 to 20,000 eggs a day. Estimates of the duration of the life of this species vary from five to seventeen years.

Calculations like these of the total number of eggs produced by parasitic worms must, however, be considered in relation to other factors. It is known, for instance, that the host exerts a considerable influence on the number of fertilized eggs produced. Particular species produce larger numbers of eggs in their usual hosts than they do in unusual hosts. It is known also that roundworms, at any rate, show a decline in the number of eggs produced as the age of the worms increase. Palmer (1955) found that an unknown number of individuals of *Necator americanus* were producing, by the eleventh month after a man had become infected with them, 799,300 eggs per day and that this level of egg-production rose gradually until, after being parasitic in the same white male person for five years, these worms were producing 1,100,100 eggs per day. The egg-production then fell gradually until, after having infected this same person for about six years, the worms were producing 731,000 eggs per day. Thereafter the egg-production gradually fell until, when·the fection had lasted in this person fifteen years, the worms were producing no eggs at all.

This rise and ultimate fall of the egg-production occurs in many species of roundworms and no doubt in many other kinds of parasitic animals. In some of the roundworms parasitic in domesticated animals there are seasonal variations of the egg-production as well, an increased number of eggs being produced in the spring. Because each of the eggs produced is capable of giving origin to an infective larva of the worm, a seasonal variation in the egg-production has an important influence on the spread of these worms among their hosts and on their capacity for causing serious disease at certain times of the year. Egg-production is also related to the number of worms required to produce disease in any host. A calculation that throws light upon this is the estimate made by American experts that 500 human hookworms must suck the blood of man for several months before severe hookworm disease is caused. If this is so, we must conclude that, if we assume, as we reasonably may, that half of these 500 hookworms are females, the minimum number of eggs passed out each day in the excreta of a person suffering from severe hookworm disease is, if we take the lowest estimate of the egg-production of *Ancylostoma duodenale* given above, $250 \times 25,000$ or about 6 million eggs. The number of eggs passed out each day by a person infected with *Necator americanus* would be proportionately smaller.

If these numbers of eggs, each one of which can potentially give rise to one infective larva of a hookworm, seem to ensure formidable degrees of infection of human beings, it is comforting to remember that roundworms are unisexual worms and that each infective larva can therefore give origin to a male or a female, not to both, and that no fertilized eggs can be produced unless both male and female worms succeed in entering and establishing themselves in a host. More comforting still is the knowledge that it has been estimated that the chances against both a male and female hookworm getting into the same host and reproducing inside it are about 18 million to 1. It is therefore clear that large numbers of both male and female hookworms, and no doubt large numbers of the males and females of other species of roundworms as well, must fail to produce fertilized eggs, even after they have successfully established themselves inside a host. This does not, of course, prevent them from sucking blood and causing disease, but it does limit their capacity to reproduce the species and provide for its survival and no doubt it is a powerful reason why these worms produce such enormous numbers of fertilized eggs. Similar facts relating to other species of parasitic worms are known and no doubt the same factors operate upon them all.

When, however, we turn to the parasitic insects and arachnids, we find that the number of eggs produced is not so large. It was explained in chapter 10, for instance, that the human lice produce not more than 50 to 300 eggs during their lives and other species of parasitic insects also produce relatively few eggs. Some of the parasitic arachnids, such as the ticks, are more prolific than this. The female *Ixodes ricinus*, for instance, which is the tick commonly found on sheep and other mammals in Britain, lays 500 to 2,000 eggs all in one batch just before she dies. Soft ticks, on the other hand, lay eggs at intervals during their lives, usually just after a meal of blood.

Perhaps the species of parasitic animals which produce the smallest numbers of offspring are those which lay, not eggs, but larvae which have been nourished inside the womb of the parasitic animal. Each tsetse fly, for instance, produces only 12 to 14 larvae during her lifetime. This reduction of the numbers of the offspring is, no doubt, associated with the necessity of nourishing the offspring one at a time inside the body of the parent and also with the elimination of the risks run by the offspring during the earliest phases of their lives.

(2) *Helping the Fertilization of the Eggs.* Among the species described in this book the unisexual blood flukes and the hookworms show clear adaptations towards helping the fertilization of the eggs. The males of the blood-flukes belonging to the genus *Schistosoma* described in chapter 5 have, as most other flukes have, relatively broad and flattened bodies, but the sides of their bodies are curled over to form a groove inside which the female worm, which has a cylindrical body adapted to life in the narrow lymphatic channels in which these flukes live, is firmly held while copulation is in progress. At other times the males and females may live separately.

The males of the hookworms show a different kind of adaptation which helps the fertilization of the eggs. They belong to the order of roundworms called the Strongyloidea, all the males of which have, at their posterior ends, an umbrella-shaped expansion of the cuticle supported by rays of stiffer material, which is applied to the genital opening of the female so that the two worms remain attached together while copulation occurs. The well-known gapeworm of poultry, *Syngamus trachea* (fig. 67), which lives in the air-passages of the fowl and other birds, and includes among its relatives one species, *Syngamus laryngeus*, which may be an accidental parasite of man, retains this form of association of the male and female worm throughout life, the smaller male being attached permanently to the region of the genital opening of the female, which is in the anterior third of her body, so that the two worms together have the shape of the letter Y, one short arm of which represents the male.

Among animals parasitic, not in man, but in other hosts, there are many interesting adaptations which help the fertilization of the eggs. Attachment of the male to the female may,

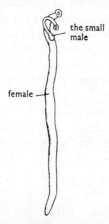

the small
male

female

Fig. 67. The gapeworm of poultry, *Syngamus trachea*, showing the small male permanently attached to the larger female

for instance, be accompanied by differences in structure of the males and females (sexual dimorphism), the structure of either the males or the females being simplified; or the females become mere bags of eggs to which the males are attached; or the males are very small and are attached to the females or to hermaphrodite individuals. The small male of the roundworm *Trichosomoides crassicauda* is actually parasitic inside the womb (*uterus*) of the female of this species.

The mention of hermaphroditism introduces the question

whether the development of both male and female sexual organs inside the same individual can be regarded as being an adaptation that helps fertilization of the eggs of parasitic animals. Hermaphroditism can hardly be an adaptation to parasitic life, because it occurs among non-parasitic animals and is, on the whole, more closely related to sedentary or inactive life than to parasitism. Among the non-parasitic Crustacea, for instance, most of the barnacles (Cirripedia) are hermaphrodite and these are sedentary organisms. Hermaphroditism also occurs among parasitic species, the adults of which are relatively inactive, such as the flukes and tapeworms, the adult phases of which are attached to their hosts by hooks and suckers. The relative inactivity of flukes and tapeworms is characteristic, in fact, not only of their adult phases, but of their larval phases as well, the whole life history tending to be passive. Hermaphroditism also occurs among species not parasitic in man which have lost, as a result of their parasitism, their limbs or other locomotor organs, so that they are relatively inactive.

Whether the occurrence of both male and female sexual organs in the same individual helps the fertilization of the eggs is more debatable. Frequently, as in the tapeworms, for instance, the male sexual organs develop and mature before the female ones do and they may have disappeared before the eggs are ready to be fertilized, a difficulty that is commonly overcome by the development of receptacles into which the sperms are introduced and stored until they are required; but the basic necessity of sexual reproduction, the need for the exchange of reproductive cells between two different individuals, must also be met, if the species is to survive and remain vigorous and capable of responding successfully to the challenges of the environment. Cross-fertilization, even among hermaphrodite individuals, is therefore necessary, at any rate, at times; and we know that it occurs. If cross-fertilization is essential, it is no great advantage to have both sexes in the same individual. This may even be, under certain circumstances, a handicap. The fact remains, however, that, among animals parasitic in man at any rate, the hermaphrodite tapeworms excel the

other species in the number of fertilized eggs that they produce. They are, in fact, rivalled only by some, but not by any
means by all, of the species of the unisexual roundworms.

All the modifications of reproductive processes so far considered in this chapter have been modifications of sexual reproduction. No mention has yet been made of species which
pass all their lives without the occurrence of any sexual process. Species of this type rely for the propagation of their
species on asexual division of individuals of the species into
two new individuals. This method is employed especially by
species the structure of which is so simple that division into
two new individuals can be accomplished. It is confined, among
parasitic animals, to the Protozoa. The division may be, as it is
among the trypanosomes, division of each individual into two
descendants only (*binary fission*), or it may be, as it is among
the malarial parasites, simultaneous division into a number of
individuals (*schizogony*). Asexual division may be the only
method of multiplication of the number of individuals, as it is
in the life histories of *Entamoeba histolytica* and the trypanosomes, or it may be combined with sexual reproduction, as it
is in the life histories of the malarial parasites. When both
asexual multiplication and sexual reproduction occur, there
may be an alternation of a number of asexual generations with
a single generation sexually produced and this may be associated, as it is in the life histories of the human malarial parasites, with an alternation of intermediate and final hosts, the
asexual multiplication occurring in the intermediate host and
the sexual reproduction in the final host.

The capacity of some species to increase their numbers by
asexual multiplication is remarkable. Among the species described in this book it is well exemplified by the human malarial parasites. The multiplication of the numbers of individuals of these species begins (cf. fig. 40) during the lives of
these parasites in the mosquitoes which are their final hosts.
As soon as the female gamete is fertilized, she becomes the
zygote, which is the exact equivalent of the fertilized egg of
more highly-organized animals. The zygote then produces,
by division of its body, the *sporoblasts*, and these produce, by

repeated division of the nucleus of each sporoblast, the *sporo-zoites*, which are the infective phases. These migrate to the salivary glands of the mosquito and 200,000 of them may be produced in a single mosquito.

These are not all the products of a single zygote, because there may be as many as 50 oocysts on the walls of a single mosquito's stomach, though the number of them is usually less than this. It is evident, nevertheless, that each zygote of the malarial parasites produces a remarkable number of infective phases.

This, however, is not by any means the full extent of the multiplication of the number of individuals that occurs. It represents only the multiplication that occurs in the final host. In the intermediate host, man, a much greater multiplication of the number of individuals takes place and this second phase of multiplication in the intermediate host may be compared with the multiplication of the number of individuals that occurs in the life histories of the flukes described above.

First, inside the cells of the liver of man, into which the sporozoites penetrate, a phase of multiple division (*schizo-gony*) occurs. *Plasmodium vivax*, may, during this phase of the infection, produce about 1,000 merozoites, each of which can infect a red blood cell; and ultimately about 1 per cent of the total number of red blood cells in the body may become infected. *Plasmodium falciparum*, however, may produce very much larger numbers of individuals. Each individual of this species may produce, during its multiplication in the cells of the liver, 40,000 merozoites, each of which can infect a red blood cell. Inside each of the infected red blood cells each schizogony produces only about 12 merozoites, but repetition of schizogony inside these cells may, if it is not checked, go on until there are 500,000 individual parasites in each cubic milli-metre of blood and some 10 to 20 per cent of the total number of red blood cells are infected. What does this phrase '10 to 20 per cent of the total number of red blood cells' mean?

Its meaning may be deduced from the facts that a healthy person has about 6 litres (6,000 cubic centimetres) of blood and that each cubic *millimetre* of blood contains about 5 million red blood cells. There are 1,000 cubic millimetres in one cubic centimetre, so that there are $1,000 \times 6,000$ cubic millimetres of blood in a healthy person and each of these contains about 5 million red blood cells. The total number of red blood cells is therefore about 5×6 million $= 30$ million million. If 10 to 20 per cent of these are infected by malarial parasites, about 3 to 6 million million malarial parasites will be present. As chapter 8 explains, the numbers of the other species of the malarial parasites may be less, because fewer merozoites are produced. *Plasmodium vivax*, for instance, produces the smaller numbers of merozoites mentioned above. Its powers of multiplication are, nevertheless, formidable. Symptoms of malaria appear when there are about 1,000 million parasites present in the host.

The flukes and tapeworms, which, like the malarial parasites, combine the alternation of asexually and sexually produced generations with alternations of intermediate and final hosts, also multiply the numbers of individuals of the species, but the multiplication takes the form, not of binary or multiple fission, but of an increase in the number of individuals derived from each fertilized egg. Whereas, for instance, each fertilized egg of a roundworm, such as the human hookworm, can produce only one larval phase, which can become only one male, or one female, adult worm, each fertilized egg of the large intestinal fluke, *Fasciolopsis buski*, described in chapter 5, gives rise to a single larval phase, the miracidium, from which arise, inside the snail intermediate host, a large number of larval phases, which culminate in numerous infective cercariae, each of which can become an adult fluke. The capacity of the species to infect the host, and therefore its ability to survive, are in this manner increased. The large intestinal fluke, for instance, produces 25,000 eggs a day and each of these eggs gives origin to numerous infective cercariae. The fact that each miracidium of the human blood-fluke, *Schistosoma mansoni*, which may live in man for 30 to 40 years, may give origin to 100,000 to 250,000 infective cercariae has been explained in chapter 5. Possibly the production of this prodigious number of cercariae is associated with the fact that species of the genus *Schistosoma*

269

are, like the roundworms, unisexual, so that each cercaria must become, not a hermaphrodite individual, but either a female or a male, and the female must meet, and be fertilized by, a male, before more fertilized eggs can be produced.

Other examples could be given of the multiplication of the number of individuals derived from a single fertilized female gamete, but enough has been said to show that this process is an important means by which the parasitic animal may not only increase its chances of infecting the host, but may also insure itself against the destruction of the individuals of its species. This process of multiplication has, on the other hand, some disadvantages for the parasitic animal. It may, for instance, produce so many parasitic individuals that the host suffers severely and may be killed, so that the parasites die with it.

The species that have indirect life histories usually affect their final hosts more severely than their intermediate hosts; but intermediate hosts, when they are heavily infected by the larval phases of these species, may also suffer disease that may be serious or even fatal. Thus man, when he is heavily infected with malarial parasites, may be very ill or he may die; and when he is infected with the cysticerci of the pork tapeworm, or with coenurus or hydatid cysts, the effects may be serious. Even the snails that are the intermediate hosts of flukes may be killed by the larval phases of the flukes that develop in them, although usually they can survive heavy infections with these phases.

CHAPTER TWELVE

Host versus Parasite

THE age-old battle of man with the parasitic animals that have always plagued him is part of the widespread battle that all kinds of hosts wage continually against their parasites. The sheep, cattle, and other domesticated animals on our farms, the birds in the air, the fishes in the rivers and seas – all kinds of animals – are bothered, in one way or another, by parasitic animals. Many plants are bothered by them too. The bugs, green flies, sawflies, mites, eelworms, and other species that damage the crops and stored products of man are too well known to need further reference here. Nor are the parasitic animals themselves free from other parasitic animals (hyperparasites) that live on them; man, in fact, has tried to use these hyperparasites to control some of the parasitic animals that injure the products of his civilization. This book, therefore, which considers only the animals that are parasitic in man himself, deals only with one facet of a warfare that goes on throughout the world of living organisms. And it is a war. Because no host, whether it be a plant or an animal, welcomes the parasite that invades it and seeks to get from it the food that it needs. The host reacts against these living invaders, just as it reacts against a splinter of wood or metal, a chemical substance or any other inanimate thing that gets into its tissues. How does it react? To some degree this depends on whether the invader is a plant or an animal. In this chapter we shall discuss more particularly how man reacts. His reactions are not basically different from those of other kinds of animals, except that the human brain enables man to devise intelligent methods of combating parasitic animals that are based on the knowledge of their structure, biology, and life histories that he has laboriously acquired. In general his reactions may be

271

classified as reactions of his tissues, reactions which take the form of the development of an immunity (resistance) against the parasitic animal and methods of attack devised by man on the parasitic animals which seek to destroy them in his body or to prevent the parasitic animals from getting into it. It is not possible in a book of this length to give more than a very brief account of the tissue reactions that are provoked in the host by parasitic animals, nor to give more than an outline of the immunity to them that many hosts develop; these are similar to the tissue reactions and immunity provoked by bacteria and viruses; but more can be said about the methods man uses to prevent them getting into his body.

Tissue Reactions

When parasitic animals enter the body of a host, or injure in any way its surface, the tissues of the host react in much the same way as they do to any other kind of invader of the body. An attempt is made to repair the damage done, or to limit the spread of irritation of the tissues caused and this response of the host expresses itself in the form of what we call an *inflammation* of the tissues concerned. More blood is sent to the site of the injury and this brings plagocytic cells which attack the invader and other cells which lay down fibrous tissue which walls off the bridgehead occupied by the parasite. If the injury is severe, or if the parasitic animal secretes or excretes into the host very irritating substances, the inflammation caused is *acute*. The part affected becomes hot, reddened and painful and lymph exuding from the blood vessels that supply it may cause it to swell up. If bacteria are introduced into it, these may add to the severity of the reaction and a septic sore or an abscess may result. This may happen even when the injury done by the parasitic animal is only relatively slight, as the surface injuries inflicted by blood-sucking fleas or horse flies, for example, are; but injuries of this kind cause itching and the person bitten scratches and introduces bacteria which cause more trouble than the parasitic animal did. In other instances the parasitic animal itself injects into the host irritating substances which are the chief cause of the reaction of the host.

Inflammation caused by parasitic animals frequently is, on the other hand, not acute; it has the slower course of the form of inflammation called *chronic* inflammation; or the reaction of the host begins as a transient acute inflammation which settles down into a chronic one. Chronic inflammation usually results in the formation by the host of fibrous tissue around the invading parasitic animal, which walls off the invader and, if it is successful, encloses it in a capsule of firmer tissues, so that the type of reaction called a *nodule* develops. The nodules characteristic of the disease caused by the filarial roundworm *Ouchocerca volvulus* described in chapter 5 are formed in this way. There are, of course, innumerable variations of these two chief forms of inflammation. Different kinds of parasitic animals tend to cause either the acute or the chronic form.

In addition to various forms of inflammation parasitic animals may cause derangements of the normal growth of the tissues of the host. They may cause it to produce excessive amounts of particular tissues (*hyperplasia*) or increase in the size of the cells of a particular tissue or of a whole organ (*hypertrophy*), an example of which is the enlargement of the spleen in malaria; or they may cause the type of cells characteristic of particular tissues to change to other types of cell (*metaplasia*); when, for instance, the lungs of man are infected with the Oriental lung fluke, *Paragonimus westermanii*, the cylindrical cells that line the smaller air-tubes (bronchioles) become, in the neighbourhood of these flukes, flattened cells more like those on the surface of the skin. Some parasitic animals may cause *neoplasia*, a term which means the formation of definite tumours, tumours being new growths of existing tissues, which perform no useful purpose; tumours go on growing independently of the control of growth that is exercised by the organism as a whole and they may be simple (benign) or malignant. Benign tumours do not reproduce themselves elsewhere in the organism, but they may exert pressure and have other effects on tissues or organs among which they grow. The hyperplasia caused by the blood fluke of man, *Schistosoma mansoni,* may, for instance, cause finger-like growths (*papillomata*) of the walls of the large intestine and *S. haematobium* may cause similar growths of the wall of the bladder; and other species of parasitic animals may cause benign tumours of various glands. Malignant tumours, such as cancer, on the other hand, can, if portions of them are detached and settle elsewhere in the body, form new tumours (*metastases; metastatic growths*) in these places. The effects of malignant tumours are always serious and frequently they are fatal. Not many parasitic animals are able to cause them, but cancer of the liver has been attributed to the Oriental liver fluke, *Opisthorchis sinensis,* and to its relative, *O. felineus,* and cancer of the bladder of man to the urinary blood-fluke, *Schistosoma haematobium;* there are instances among hosts other than man.

IMMUNITY (RESISTANCE) TO PARASITIC ANIMALS

In a book of this size this complex subject cannot be discussed in detail. Fuller accounts are given by Chandler (1955), Craig and Faust (1955), Belding (1952), and Lapage (1951). Here there is space to say that immunity plays an important part in the defence of the host against all kinds of parasitic organisms, parasitic animals included. It is a response of the whole host acting as a unified, integrated organism, so that, although it may, in some instances, be a response of the tissues at the site at which the invading organism damages the body of the host, so that we can speak of a *local immunity,* it usually also affects organs distant from the site of this local injury. It provokes, that is to say, certain organs of the host to produce substances called *antibodies,* which circulate in the host's blood and combat the invader. Each species of invading organism calls forth the production of antibodies that operate either only, or most strongly, against itself, or only against itself and its nearest relatives, so that the antibodies are specific to each species of invader. Antibodies produced against parasitic animals are, however, not so specific as those produced against bacteria and the other organisms generally known as microbes. The immunity developed against parasitic animals is, nevertheless, not basically different from the immunity developed against microbes and it falls into the same categories. It may be natural or acquired.

The term *natural* (innate) *immunity* (resistance) means that an invading organism, whether it is a parasitic animal, virus, or one of the bacteria, cannot infect a host that is naturally immune to it, even when it has the opportunity to do so. Man, for example, cannot be infected by the roundworms parasitic in the dog, although he can be infected by the tapeworms of the dog described in chapter 6, to which he is not naturally immune. Before, however, we can decide that the host is, in fact, naturally immune, it is essential to fulfil the proviso that the parasitic organism must have the opportunity to infect the supposedly naturally immune host. We must not, for example, conclude that man is naturally immune to infection with the trypanosomes that cause sleeping sickness, merely because these organisms are not found in him in Britain or India. Man is immune in these countries merely because these trypanosomes have no opportunity to infect him in these places. As soon as he goes to Africa and exposes himself to infection through tsetse flies there, the Englishman may become infected and then he will show that he is not naturally immune. He may, in fact, be more susceptible to these particular organisms than his brothers and sisters in Africa who have been exposed all their lives to this infection and have therefore acquired a degree of immunity to it.

Acquired Immunity may be either active or passive. Active acquired immunity is always the result of an active response made by the host. It may be *natural* and it is then the result of an infection naturally acquired during the host's normal life. Man, for example, develops an active acquired immunity to malaria as a result of infection with malarial parasites naturally acquired.

Active acquired immunity may, on the other hand, be *artificial*. It is then an active response by the host produced by the artificial introduction into man of living or dead organisms in the form of vaccines, which make the host *actively* produce antibodies against these organisms. This happens, for example, when people are vaccinated against smallpox. The host gets a mild attack of the disease and produces antibodies against it which protect the host against it for years or even for the rest of its life. Unfortunately we cannot use this most valuable form of immunity to protect man against parasitic animals that infect him, though it is used for the protection of some of our domesticated animals against some of the parasitic animals that infect them; it is used, for instance, to protect cattle against the Protozoa that cause the serious and often fatal disease called redwater fever.

Passive acquired immunity is never an active response by the host. It is always the result of introduction into the host of antibodies prepared in the body of some other host. It is always weaker than active acquired immunity and does not last so long. Passive acquired immunity may be conferred on a host in two chief ways. It may be conferred by a mammalian mother on the child in her womb. When this happens, the mother passes on antibodies produced in her own blood to the young in the womb by way of the blood circulating through the placenta; or she may, in a few instances, pass them on in the earliest secretion of her milk glands, which is called the colostrum, or in the milk which comes later. Passive immunity acquired in this manner by the young is naturally acquired. Passive immunity may, on the other hand, be conferred by man on any host, young or older, when he introduces into that host antibodies, or substances called antitoxins, which neutralize the poisons produced by the parasitic organisms. Passive immunity acquired in this manner is artificially acquired.

Unfortunately the methods just described of conferring immunity *artificially* on the host cannot yet be used effectively against the animals that may be parasitic in man. The bacteriologist can devise vaccines, sera, and antitoxins for use in this manner against parasitic bacteria, but corresponding vaccines and sera cannot be made for use against parasitic animals, largely because the antibodies produced against parasitic animals are not so specific as those that the hosts produce against bacteria. For much the same reason the skin-tests and other serological tests which bacteriologists use so successfully for finding out whether a particular organism is present in a host, or whether it has been present in the past, are not so useful for the detection of infections with parasitic animals. For the diagnosis of infections with some species of parasitic animals, however, they can be used. Thus fluid taken from hydatid cysts will, if it is injected into the skin of a person who has one or more of these cysts in the body, cause the formation of a wheal on the skin which is not produced on the skin of an uninfected person. A promising recent development in the immunology of parasitic infections is, moreover, the discovery by veterinarians that vaccines made by Roentgen-ray irradiation of the infective larvae of roundworms parasitic in cattle and dogs will confer considerable immunity on these hosts and it is likely that important progress will be made in the comparatively near future in the control and treatment of parasitic infections, especially those due to parasitic worms, by serological methods.

Immunity to parasitic animals plays an important part in preventing or lessening their effects on the host and in limiting the spread of the harm done to the host. For this reason the treatment of infections with parasitic animals, and plans devised for the control of infections with them, include measures designed to maintain at its highest level any immunity that may be developed. All forms of immunity are, for instance, undermined by malnutrition or the effects of other diseases. Good nutrition, therefore, by which is meant not the quantity of the food, but its quality, its content of mineral elements, fats, carbohydrates, proteins and, especially, of vitamins, is essential for the maintenance of immunity. This is especially true in the tropical parts of the world, in which the most injurious species of parasitic animals are especially prevalent and in which malnutrition may be one of the most serious afflictions of man.

THE CONTROL OF INFECTIONS WITH PARASITIC ANIMALS

This extensive subject, an adequate consideration of which might fill the whole of this book, is, in effect, the prerogative of man. It is true that some other animals seem to the human observer to try to avoid infection with some species of parasitic animals. Cattle, for instance, seem to try to avoid the warble flies, and sheep make the most vigorous efforts to avoid giving to the sheep nasal flies any opportunity to deposit their parasitic larvae in the nostrils of the sheep; but man alone has been able to devise extensive, costly, and elaborate methods of controlling infections with the parasitic animals that cause him so much suffering and inflict on him so much economic loss. These methods of control are all based on the detailed knowledge of the structure, biology, and life histories of these parasitic animals that devoted men and women have accumulated by years of patient study and at the cost of great sacrifices made by the students themselves. We can divide the measures of control that are used into those that are directed against the adult parasitic animals while they are inside or on the surface of the human body and those that are designed to prevent the entry of the infective phases into man.

With the former category of measures of control this book is not concerned. They include the administration by medical men of drugs that kill the adult parasitic animals and accounts of these drugs are given in some of the books mentioned in the bibliography at the end of this book. They include various substances, called anthelmintics, which are used to kill parasitic worms, the antimalarial drugs and the modern remedies for infections with trypanosomes that are so successful and the insecticides and acaricides, such as DDT, benzene hexachloride and related substances, which are successfully used to kill such adult parasitic animals as the mosquitoes, tsetse flies, lice, fleas, bugs, and the mites which cause scabies, which in themselves may not all cause serious human disease but are important because they transmit to man parasitic animals that do cause serious or fatal illness. Most of the drugs or insecticides or acaricides thus used are dangerous and must be used with care and under the supervision of experts who know the risks involved and the precautions that must be taken.

The second group of control measures, the group that includes the measures designed to prevent the infection of man, is also the concern of the expert in the sense that these measures are based on expert knowledge of the life histories and biology of the parasitic animals concerned; but it also involves the details of the lives of human beings in all the countries of the world and is therefore a matter of public interest. The personal habits of individuals are involved, as well as racial habits or customs, the means we employ for travelling about the world, our methods of taking food and drink, and sometimes our religious practices, so that the control of infection with parasitic animals is unfortunately bound up with the social, industrial, or even with the political and military activities of man. The accounts of the life histories of parasitic animals given in the preceding chapters should have made this clear. To make it clearer still some methods used for the control of infection with particular species of parasitic animals will now be briefly described. They can be divided into methods directed against species that infect man through the mouth and those that are directed against species that infect him through the skin or by other routes.

Control of Infection through the Mouth

Most parasitic animals use this route of entry into the host and the host conveys the infection phase of the parasitic animal to the mouth either in its food or drink or by means of the hands or of implements introduced for various reasons into the mouth. The infective phases thus conveyed to the mouth are either (1) cysts, such as those of *Entamoeba histolytica* or those containing the cercariae of such flukes as the large intestinal fluke, *Fasciolopsis buski*; or eggs containing an infective larva, such as those of *Ascaris lumbricoides* or the human threadworm, *Enterobius vermicularis*; or (2) the infective larvae which enter, in the course of the life history of the parasitic animal, food which man eats; this group includes such infective larvae as those of the trichina worm, *Trichinella spiralis*, which has a direct life history, and those of species with indirect life histories which enter intermediate hosts which are eaten by man, such as the larvae of the Guinea worm, *Dracunculus medinensis* or those of the beef tapeworm, *Taenia saginata*, and the pork

279

tapeworm, *Taenia solium*, or those of the fish tapeworm contained in fish and those of the Oriental lung and liver flukes contained in fishes or crayfishes and crabs respectively.

(1) The control of infection by means of cysts, infective eggs, and similar phases of the parasitic animal that are protected in resistant envelopes is not so easy as it may seem to be and may be, in some instances, impossible.

All these phases come from the faeces of man or other animals and to civilized peoples it may seem possible to protect human food and drink from contamination with these excreta. Efficient sanitation and efficient disposal of sewage certainly go a long way towards the control of infections conveyed in this manner. They protect human food and drink from contamination with human excreta at any rate. They may, however, break down. One outbreak of amoebic dysentery, for instance, that occurred among the residents in a first-class American hotel was due to a fault in the water-system which enabled the effluent from the lavatories to overflow temporarily into the supply of drinking water.

It might be thought also that modern methods of sewage disposal would kill all the eggs of *Ascaris lumbricoides* present in human excreta, even though these eggs are among the most resistant of all the non-parasitic phases of parasitic animals. The processes to which these eggs are subjected in sewage disposal units do, in fact, destroy large numbers of these eggs; but workers in Germany and Russia have shown that considerable numbers of these eggs may, nevertheless, be still alive when they pass out in the sewage effluent and that, when this effluent is used to water salad plants that are eaten uncooked by man, the surviving eggs may get on to these plants and may then infect people who eat the salad plants. This actually happened in Odessa and Moscow. Another striking instance of it was discovered in a German city in which more than half the population were infected with *Ascaris lumbricoides*. When the cause of this high incidence of infection was investigated, it was found that eggs of *Ascaris lumbricoides*, present in human excreta from this city, were escaping alive in the sewage effluent and this effluent was being conducted out to a village near by and used there to water the market-gardens from which the city derived most of its supply of salad plants. *Ascaris lumbricoides* was in this manner being conducted continually from the people in the city to the salad plants that they ate uncooked, so that they were continually re-infecting themselves. The inhabitants of the village in which the salad plants were grown were also eating these plants uncooked and an even higher percentage of them were infected with *Ascaris*.

The remedy for this kind of infection is, of course, improvement of the methods of disposal of the sewage and prevention of its use for watering plants that are eaten uncooked. Washing the plants before they are eaten will no doubt remove some of the eggs on them, but it cannot be relied upon to remove them all. The same is true of fruits, such as strawberries, which can, it is known, convey infection with *Ascaris lumbricoides*. The eggs of this species may, in fact, be so numerous in some parts of the world that it may be impossible to make sure that they are excluded from all forms of human food or drink.

The same considerations apply to such infective phases as the cysts of *Entamoeba histolytica*, although these are less resistant to such factors as drying, cold, the high temperatures and sunlight of tropical countries, and other physical factors that operate upon them once they have left the host. Even less resistant to these factors are the eggs of the human threadworm, *Enterobius vermicularis*; but the high incidence of this species in man all over the world shows that this worm is not unduly handicapped by the relatively feeble resistance of its infective eggs. The stickiness of these eggs and the advantages this confers upon them have been already discussed in chapter 4.

The two species just considered are practically confined to man, so that human excreta are the only sources of infection with them that need be considered. When, however, a species is parasitic in hosts other than man, protection of human food and drink against the excreta of these hosts is also necessary. The problem is then more difficult; it may indeed, be impossible to prevent infective phases from getting into human food and drink and the only effective method of control is to cook solid foods sufficiently to kill infective phases in it and to boil all water that is drunk.

The examples so far considered illustrate methods which seek to prevent the infection of man with the infective phases of the parasitic animal which become adult parasites in man. But man may swallow the eggs of some species of parasitic animals which may then become larvae in him, so that man becomes the intermediate host. This may happen, for instance, if he swallows the eggs of *Taenia solium*, the pork tapeworm, or those of the hydatid tapeworm of the dog, *Echinococcus granulosus*. The eggs of *Taenia solium*, if man ingests them, become cysticerci in him and may cause the serious disease *cysticercosis*, mentioned in chapter 6. The eggs of the hydatid tapeworm of the dog, if man ingests them, become hydatid cysts in the human body. It is hardly ever possible, even in highly-civilized societies, to make sure that all foods eaten uncooked by man, such as salad plants grown in allotments and gardens, are not contaminated by the excreta of dogs. We can, on the other hand, take precautions against infecting ourselves with the eggs of the hydatid tapeworm which may get on to the hairy coats of dogs, or into its mouth and may then be transferred to the hands of human beings, especially perhaps to those of children or of adults who pet and fondle their dogs or allow them to lick their faces or the plates from which they feed, with the result that the eggs may be swallowed to become, in the human body, hydatid cysts.

In other instances the control of infection through the mouth is designed to prevent the eggs of the parasitic animal from entering through the mouth, not of man, but of an intermediate host that is eaten by man. This is, for instance, one of the methods by which man seeks to prevent infection of himself with the beef tapeworm. He tries to prevent the eggs of this species from getting into the food of the cattle that are the intermediate hosts. These eggs, may, as those of *Ascaris lumbricoides* can, survive through the processes to which they are subjected in the course of sewage disposal and they may then be carried alive, by birds, or by streams polluted by sewage effluent, or by sewage products used to irrigate or manure pastures, to the grazing-grounds of beef cattle, which may then swallow the eggs and become infected with cysticerci. Man can, if he likes, guard against these risks; and he can also forbid the deposit of human excreta on such pastures. The other methods that he takes to guard himself against cysticerci that may, in spite of the precautions just mentioned, get into beef that he eats, are described below.

(2) We may turn now to means of control that are directed, not against the entry of the eggs or cysts of the parasitic animal through the human mouth, but against the entry of its infective larvae through this portal into the human body. The cercarial larvae of the blood flukes and the infective larvae of hookworms may, for instance, enter by this route, although they usually enter by penetrating the skin. A species that invariably infects man by the entry of its infective larvae through the mouth is the trichina worm, *Trichinella spiralis*, described in chapter 4. These larvae are, it will be remembered, in the muscles of its hosts and man usually infects himself by eating pig-meat infected with these larvae. Serious epidemics of the disease (trichiniasis) caused by this worm have, however, resulted from human consumption of the infected flesh of other hosts of this roundworm. In Germany, for instance, one epidemic was caused by eating bear meat infected with the larvae of *T. spiralis* and in Greenland man has been infected by eating the flesh of the polar bear, walrus, and seal. The dogs in Greenland are often also infected by the meat of these animals, on which they are fed. In most countries, however, the pig is the usual source of the infection and control measures are directed entirely against this animal. They attempt to prevent (a) the infection of the pig; (b) the infection of man.

(a) Pigs usually infect themselves by eating rats infected with the trichina worm that get into their styes or by eating infected meat on which the pigs are fed. Infection of the pigs by the latter method can be prevented by rearing pigs entirely on grain meal or by cooking all food given to them that contains either meat or offal derived from animals. This is, in fact, successfully done, and nowadays well-balanced rations are available for pigs that are processed so thoroughly that the larvae of the trichina worm could not possibly survive in them. The prevention of the entry of rats into quarters occupied by pigs is difficult and frequently impossible, but it is important to try to keep out the rats, because even if only one pig is infected by eating an infected rat, its flesh may be mixed with that of other pigs in the making of sausages and other forms of pig-meat and these infected pork-products may be distributed among a relatively large number of people, who may all be infected in varying degrees. Because it is thus difficult to make sure that pigs are not infected with the trichina worm, control methods are in most countries rigidly applied to prevention of the infection of man.

(b) Man may prevent infection of himself by two main methods. He can adopt a system of meat-inspection which submits all carcasses of pigs to a rigid examination by experts, who take samples of the flesh, especially samples of the muscles most likely to be infected, and squeeze them flat between plates of glass and then either examine these samples under a suitable magnification for the larvae or throw the magnified images of them on to an illuminated screen. This method takes time and requires the employment of skilled inspectors. It cannot, moreover, examine all the muscles of a pig and it is always possible that it may fail to detect infections of muscles, or parts of them, that cannot be examined. For this reason, and for economic reasons also, some countries either supplement or replace this method by another one. Samples of pork, or samples of processed pig-meat, are taken and given to rats as food. After an interval long enough to enable any larvae of the trichina worm to develop into adult worms in the rats and to produce larvae that infect the rats' muscles, the rats are killed and their muscles are digested in an artificial digestive juice. The product of this digestion is then examined for the presence of the larvae of the worm. This method takes some weeks and requires even more expert technicians than direct examination of pig-meat does, but it is likely, on the whole, to detect more light infections of the pig.

A further method of prevention of the infection of man is, however, available and this is, if it is efficiently carried out, the simplest and the most efficient of all. Pig-meat, whatever form it takes, can be cooked sufficiently to kill any larvae of the worm that may be in it, or suitable refrigeration can be used to kill them. In order to make certain that the larvae will be killed, the pork must be raised to a temperature of 58·3° c. (137° f.), or it must be cooled to a temperature of *minus* 15° c. at least and this low temperature must be maintained for not less than twenty days. The maintenance of the low temperature for this period of time is important. When cooking is used to kill the larvae, it is no less important to make sure that all parts of the meat cooked are raised to the temperature stated. Ordinary kitchen cooking may raise the outer parts of a leg of pork to this temperature, but it may not kill larvae in the deeper parts of the joint and these deeper parts may be the very parts of the meat that are most relished. More than one epidemic of trichiniasis has, in fact, been caused in this way by larvae in the deeper parts of large joints that were not sufficiently cooked.

It is possible for even such relatively small quantities of pork as those contained in sausages to be cooked so lightly that the larvae are not killed in them. Some authorities, indeed, recommend that sausages should be cut in half lengthwise and that each half should be well-cooked. Certainly pork sausages are a common cause of the infection of man with these larvae. Usually they infect human beings who eat them without any cooking at all. The history of trichiniasis repeatedly shows this and it reveals the fact that numbers of people of all classes of society in various countries, among which Britain is included, prefer to eat raw pork and especially raw sausage-meat.

One outbreak of trichiniasis in England was very instructive in this respect. It was found that the people most heavily infected were the factory girls who had little time to prepare a meal to take to the factory and therefore made sandwiches of raw pork sausage-meat and ate these for lunch; their fathers, on the other hand, who had sausages for supper at night, insisted on them being well-cooked and they were therefore only lightly infected; the mothers, who cooked the sausages for their husbands, and handled them with their fingers or even tasted portions of them while they were being cooked, were more heavily infected than their husbands, but less heavily than their daughters. An instructive instance of human infection that occurred under very different circumstances, was the infection of a German commando unit operating during the Second World War on the Polish frontier. They stole a pig from a neighbouring farmer and ate its flesh raw. The result was that all of them were not long afterwards put out of action by the trichina worm.

While these two methods of preventing the infection of man with the trichina worm are the methods most often used at the present time, the development of atomic energy may provide us in the future with a third and a very efficient method. For it is now known that exposure of pork infected with the larvae of the trichina worm to the radioactivity of the products of nuclear fission will, if it is sufficiently prolonged, kill any larvae of the trichina worm in the meat and that shorter exposures to it will cause the female worms to produce larvae that are unable to develop. Experiments which are now in progress may therefore give us a new method of making sure that any larvae present in pork cannot infect man. One advantage of sterilization effected in this manner by irradiation is that it does not raise the temperature of the meat appreciably; nor need it expose people who eat the meat to any effects of irradiation. We are not yet, however, able to put this promising method into general use.

The trichina worm, although it is one of the most important of the animals parasitic in man that infect him when he eats meat, is not by any means the only species that infects man in this way. The beef and pork tapeworms also use this method, but they are species with indirect life histories of which man is the final host and man infects himself with them when he eats the intermediate host.

It will be remembered that the larval phases (*cysticerci*) of these two tapeworms wait in the muscles of the ox and pig respectively until man eats these muscles in the form of beef and pork. To guard himself from infection with them he uses two of the methods used to prevent infection with the trichina worm, namely, meat inspection and cooking and refrigeration of the meat. Meat inspection may or may not be efficient. In many countries it is; but cooking or refrigeration are more reliable. The cysticerci of the beef tapeworm are killed by cooking beef at 135° F. or more, until it is uniformly grey and its juice is no longer red, or by refrigerating it at *minus* 8° F. to minus 10° F. for ten days; pickling beef in brine will not kill the cysticerci. The cysticerci of the pork tapeworm, which are nowadays rare in pig-meat in Britain, Germany, Denmark, the United States, and Australia, are killed by cooking pork at 113 to 122° F. or refrigerating it at 14 to 18° F. for 4 days, but chilling the pork at 32° F. is not adequate. It is necessary, when cooking is relied upon, to make sure that all parts of the beef or pork reach the temperatures stated.

Among other species of parasitic animals that have indirect life histories and infect man by developing in an intermediate host that enters his mouth in his food or drink are the Guinea worm described in chapter 6 and the fish tapeworm and the Oriental lung and liver flukes described in chapter 7. The intermediate hosts of the guinea worm are freshwater Crustacea belonging to the genus *Cyclops*. Infection of man with this species can therefore be prevented by killing all the species of the genus *Cyclops*. Attempts to do this are made by treating water supplies, whether they are used for drinking or other purposes, with copper sulphate, which kills the *Cyclops*, and by introducing into the water supplies certain fish which feed on these Crustacea. Drinking water can, of course, be boiled before it is used and the people can be warned, by means of lectures and demonstrations, of the methods by which the infection is acquired. Destruction of species of the genus *Cyclops*, and of their relatives belonging to the genus *Diaptomus*, which are used by the fish tapeworm, *Diphyllobothrium latum*, as its first intermediate hosts, will also disrupt the life history of this tapeworm. These first intermediate hosts, can, of course, be infected only if the excreta of the final hosts contaminate the fresh water in which they live. Little can, however, be done to prevent this, because so many animals other than man may be the final hosts and may contaminate water supplies with their excreta. Control of the infection of man with this species usually concentrates, for these reasons, on trying to make sure that the freshwater fish that are the second intermediate hosts of this tapeworm are cooked sufficiently to kill any plerocercoid larvae that may be present in them.

The same principles apply to the control of human infections with the Oriental flukes, *Metagonimus yokogawai* and *Paragonimus westermanii* described in chapter 7. Both these species use snails as their first intermediate hosts and the measures taken against snail intermediate hosts described below may be put into action against these. It is difficult, and frequently impossible, especially in tropical countries, to destroy all the snails (cf. below). Both these species have, moreover, several final hosts, the eggs from which can infect the snails, so that there is little hope that destruction of the snails will control infection with these species. It is better to cook properly their second intermediate hosts, namely, the trout and other freshwater fish that contain the cercariae of *Metagonimus yokogawai* and the crayfishes and crabs which harbour the cercariae of *Paragonimus westermanii*. It is, of course, not easy to enforce, among Eastern peoples, a measure like this. It is especially difficult, perhaps, to prevent infection with *Paragonimus westermanii* by this method, because it is an Oriental custom to eat the crayfishes and crabs either raw or after they have been stored in brine, or made into dishes with wine. Japanese authors have shown that, when soups and other dishes are made from the crabs, the cercariae may cling to the knife used to chop up the crabs, or to the bamboo basket into which the crab's meat is put, or to the hands of the cook and may then be transferred to other foods. This is a good example of the fact that the details of the habits of peoples must be known if control is to be made effective.

The remarks made about the two species just discussed will have drawn the reader's attention to the important part that snails may play in the spread of species of parasitic animals which have indirect life histories. Snails may be either the first intermediate hosts only of such species as the Oriental flukes just discussed, or they may be the only intermediate hosts, as they are in the life histories of the common liver fluke of sheep and cattle, *Fasciola hepatica,* and its relative the large intestinal fluke, *Fasciolopsis buski* described in chapter 5. In the life histories of these two species, the cercariae which infect man leave the snails and encyst on plants and man may prevent infection of himself by not eating the plants concerned unless they have been cooked. On the comparatively rare occasions when he infects himself with the liver fluke of sheep and cattle, he does so by eating water-cress or similar plants, or even windfall fruits, such as apples, on which the cercariae have encysted.

Snails may, however, be the intermediate hosts of the blood flukes described in chapter 5 and infection with the cercariae of these flukes, while it may take place through the mouth of man when he drinks water containing them, usually occurs by penetration of human skin by the cercariae. In this respect the blood flukes resemble the hookworms, whose active, infective larvae may also infect man through the mouth, but usually penetrate his skin. We are thus introduced to the whole group of parasitic animals that infect man through his skin; and in this group we include the blood-sucking insects and other external parasites which either make the skin of man their home or feed themselves by penetrating through it.

Infection through the Skin

Parasitic animals that enter man by this route do so either by the efforts of their active infective phases which bore through the skin, or by the introduction of their infective phases through the skin by another kind of parasitic animal, which may be either a mere mechanical vector which acts as a needle or any other puncturing instrument might do, or it is a host of the parasitic animal, inside which the parasitic animal must undergo changes before it can infect man. How can man protect his skin from these invading infective phases? Let us consider the hookworm and the blood flukes first, whose infective phases penetrate human skin without the aid of any other animal. The hookworms have direct life histories, so that their infective larvae come from the eggs of the adult worms; and these are derived from human faeces only. The blood flukes have indirect life histories, so that their infective phases, which are cercariae, come from the intermediate hosts, which are aquatic snails. The snails are, however, infected by miracidial larvae which come from eggs derived from the faeces of man, although the eggs of *Schistosoma japonicum* come from other animals also.

The Control of Infections with Hookworms

Because these worms are virtually confined to man, human infection can come only from other human beings; and because the infection is effected by the non-parasitic third infective larvae derived from the eggs, which are found only in human excreta, the most effective control will be to prevent the deposition of human excreta in any situation in which they can develop and produce infective larvae that can make contact with the skin of man.

This may seem, to civilized and hygienic people, to be an easy matter; and the provision of ordinary sanitation does, in fact, prevent infection with these worms, provided that the sanitary equipment is properly used. It has eradicated these worms from places in which they used to cause much serious hookworm disease. But in some parts of the world good sanitation cannot be established. Education of the people in the method of infection, and the provision of modern hygiene have both failed; in other parts of the world lack of water has prevented the installation of water-closets and the proper use of other methods of disposal of human excreta cannot be enforced. These excreta are, in fact, often used still as manure and therefore are the means of spreading infection not only with hookworms, but with other species with direct life histories, such as *Entamoeba histolytica* and *Ascaris lumbricoides*. This practice of using human excreta as manure still occurs not only in the East where its use has long been known, but even in some European countries. The spread of hookworm infection is due, however, more often to the indiscriminate deposition of human excreta in the soil on which bare-legged and bare-footed people walk, or around the dwellings in which the people live, or on ground on which their children play, or in other places in which the people congregate. In the warm, moist soils of countries in which these habits prevail, the eggs of the hookworms readily survive and develop and these soils provide a favourable environment for the non-parasitic larvae derived from the eggs. The first larvae liberated from the eggs become infective larvae in a few days and the scantily-clothed or naked human skin offers them plenty of opportunities for penetration of it. In the cold or more temperate parts of the world these eggs and larvae cannot survive and the skin is more usually covered in these countries with boots or other coverings. For this reason the hookworms are parasites especially of the warmer parts of the world.

The remedies against infection with them are obvious. Removal by means of drugs of the adult worms, prevention of the contamination of the ground with human excreta and the protection of the skin, especially the skin of the feet, ankles, hands, and arms, should do much to free human beings from these very harmful pests.

The Control of Infection with the Blood-Flukes

The life histories of these species are indirect, and their infective phases, the skin-penetrating cercariae, come only from the snails which are the intermedite hosts. These snails are aquatic and the cercariae are also aquatic, so that the infection is always water-borne. Control of infection with these species therefore concentrates on (1) protection of the skin of man from water containing the cercariae; (2) cutting off the source of these cercariae by destroying the snails from which they come; (3) preventing the infection of the snails with larval stages of the blood-flukes by trying to avoid contamination of the waters in which these snails live with the excreta of man and other final hosts of the blood-flukes from which these larval phases are derived.

The third of these categories of control measures will vary to some extent according to the species of blood-fluke that is being controlled. *Schistosoma haematobium* and *S. mansoni* use man chiefly as their final host, so that most human infections are derived from human excreta. A good deal may therefore be done to prevent infection of the snail intermediate hosts of these two species by preventing contacts between human excreta and the water in which the snails live. *S. japonicum*, on the other hand, uses not only man, but also other mammals as its final hosts, and among these other animals are pets, such as dogs and cats and domesticated animals, and it is difficult or impossible to prevent these other hosts from fouling the waters with their excreta. Control of this species must therefore depend chiefly on the other two categories of control measures mentioned above.

Destruction of the snail intermediate hosts is based on our detailed knowledge of the biology of the species of snails involved. Experts must be employed to identify them and the pools, irrigation canals and other waterways in which they live must be cleaned and kept free from the vegetation under which the snails shelter and breed. The water itself may be treated with chemical substances, such as slaked lime, copper sulphate or copper carbonate, which kill the snails. Irrigation canals can be periodically drained and allowed to dry and this kills many snails, but many of them may survive by burrowing in the mud and taking shelter there. They may lose their infection with the larvae of the blood-flukes while they are thus sheltering, but they can survive for long periods out of water and, as soon as the water returns, they can acquire new infections and can quickly repopulate the waterways with new generations of snails.

The skin of man may be protected by wearing rubber gloves or boots and by boiling all water taken from natural sources. Drinking water should be boiled, because the cercariae can infect man through the lining of the mouth or, by swallowing the water. Adequate treatment of the water with chlorine will also kill cercariae in it. Filtration of drinking water may remove cercariae from it if the filters are adequate and the German Afrika Corps in North Africa was supplied, during the Second World War, with filters for this purpose; but it is wiser not to rely upon this method. The cercariae need only a few minutes to penetrate the skin, so that cold water taken direct from natural sources and used for cold baths, washing, and shaving is a possible source of infection. Measures such as these are, of course, possible for people who can afford the cost of them; but they can hardly be applied to the local populations of the countries in which the blood-flukes flourish. In countries such as Venezuela and Algeria, for instance, in which irrigation canals are used to water the land, these canals provide favourable conditions for the life and propagation of the snails. Children play in and around the canals, their mothers use the water for washing and the men, especially those who help to operate the irrigation systems, are continually exposing their skins to infection. Because the sanitary habits of the people are often primitive, the water is continually being contaminated with human faeces and the snails are constantly being infected. Control of the infection is, under such conditions, inevitably difficult and can hardly be more than partially effective.

The Control of Infections Transmitted by the Bites of Blood-Sucking Arthropods

The most important of the parasitic animals that are transmitted to man through his skin by blood-sucking arthropods are the trypanosomes transmitted by tsetse flies and blood-sucking bugs, the leishmanias transmitted by sandflies and the malarial parasites transmitted by mosquitoes. The other insects and the fleas, ticks, and mites described in chapter 10, which either make the human skin their home or visit it to suck blood and, when they do this, transmit to man bacteria or viruses that cause serious diseases, also come into this category, but we are not strictly concerned in this book with these, but only with the arthropods which transmit parasitic animals. The measures taken against them, however, are not widely different from those taken against the species which transmit parasitic animals. They are all based on our detailed knowledge of the life histories and biology of these arthropods. They cannot be fully described in a book of this kind. Some of the larger books and other publications devoted entirely to them are mentioned in the bibliography at the end of this book. They are, moreover, continually changing as new knowledge of the biology of the arthropods concerned and new insecticides and acaricides become available.

The control of blood-sucking insects differs, naturally, to some extent, from the control of arachnid species, such as the ticks and mites, because the life histories and biology of these two groups of arthropods differs considerably. In both groups it is usually the adult phase that sucks the blood of man and the problem of protecting man is, in some instances, complicated by the fact that the blood-sucking arthropods feed, not only on man, but on other hosts as well. Protection of man is therefore only a part of the problem and other hosts, access to which cannot be denied to the arthropods, may maintain these suckers of human blood in spite of all the measures we can take to protect human beings. This is, for instance, a difficulty experienced in the control of tsetse flies in Africa, some account of which has been given in chapter 9. It is an even greater difficulty in the control of the reduviid bugs which transmit *Trypanosoma cruzi* to man in South America, where the numerous alternative hosts of these bugs and the habits and customs of the people make it virtually impossible to prevent the bugs from having access to man. It is a difficulty also in the control of leeches, fleas, ticks, and other species, which feed on other hosts when man is not available and thus maintain themselves. The fact that the sandflies that transmit *Leishmania tropica* to man (see chapter 9) maintain themselves on the blood of rodents is a typical instance of this kind of difficulty. In this particular instance the difficulty is all the greater because the disease of the skin caused by *L. tropica* is probably, as tuberculosis of cattle and rabies of the dog and other animals also are, a *zoonosis*, that is to say, a disease of other animals the cause of which can live in, and cause disease of, man. It is therefore well established in other animals, and is, for this reason, all the more resistant to our efforts to eradicate it.

The methods used for the control of insect vectors of parasitic animals seek to attack the various phases of the life histories of these vectors. When the eggs are vulnerable, as those of the lice are, these are attacked with substances that will kill them, or the eggs of species, such as the mosquitoes, which lay their eggs in water, may be attacked by chemical substances used to kill the aquatic larvae also. The larvae of mosquitoes may be attacked with Paris Green and other substances distributed by hand or by other means in their aquatic breeding places. The larvae of horse flies, clegs, Mango, and other tabanid flies, which are also aquatic and typically live in water throughout the winter, may also be killed by these substances, or they may be asphyxiated, as the larvae of mosquitoes also can be, by covering the water in which they live with a layer of oil, so that they are denied access to the air that they must breathe. The larvae of other species of insects are attacked with insecticides applied to places in which they breed. The nymphs of ticks and mites are attacked in the same way. The pupae of insects cannot usually be satisfactorily attacked, but good results have followed the collection and destruction of the pupae of tsetse flies, which lay, not eggs, but larvae that almost immediately pupate, so that the pupa is the only larval phase available for attack.

Attacks on the adult phases are, when man is the host, in many respects easier, because man collects the arthropods on his body or in his clothes and thus concentrates them in a limited area. Chemical substances, called *repellents*, which discourage the arthropods from using man as a host, may be used; they may be effective against some species of insects, but are useless against others, such as the sandflies. The sandflies also evade such measures as protective screens, mosquito-nets and similar contrivances designed to keep blood-sucking insects away from man, because the sandflies are small enough to get through the meshes of these screens. Against mosquitoes and tsetse flies, however, nets and other kinds of screens can be useful.

The main attack on the adult phases, however, whether they are insects, ticks, or mites, is nowadays made with insecticides and acaricides. Lice may be killed by the application of these to the bodies of people infected with these insects, and they may be applied to the bodies of the hosts of ticks and mites. They are useful also for the control of the maggots described in chapter 10, which attack the skin and cause myiasis. The most remarkable method of controlling maggots which cause this disease is, however, the method recently used to eradicate the maggots of *Callitroga hominivorax* from Florida. The basis of this method was the fact that these flies mate only once a year and American workers conceived the idea of breeding enormous numbers of male flies which had been sterilized by irradiation and releasing them over the area affected, in the hope that they would mate with the female flies with the result that no larvae (maggots) would be produced. The experiment involved the breeding of 50 million irradiated flies a week and the distribution of these flies by means of aeroplanes over the whole State of Florida. The experiment was brilliantly successful. This species of fly, which caused heavy losses of farm and other animals, was eradicated from the area involved.

For the control of adult mosquitoes, sand-flies, tsetse flies, and other winged insects and also for the control of the wingless fleas, the insecticides are sprayed over dwellings occupied by man or over the aeroplanes and other means of transport that man employs. The control of malaria relies nowadays mainly on this method of attacking the vectors and it is also used, as chapter 9 explains, for the control of tsetse flies. Aeroplanes may be used for spraying the insecticides over extensive tracts of country infested with these flies. Against the bed bug it is more usual to employ fumigation of the houses and furniture of people attacked by these pests. The architect and builder also help by designing buildings free from the cracks and crevices in which the bugs live. Control of the assassin bugs which transmit *Trypanosoma cruzi* in South America is more difficult, because these bugs, unlike the wingless bed bugs, can rapidly fly for considerable distances and can also move very quickly on their feet. Screens and mosquito nets would be useful against them if the huts in which the people live did not provide, in their thatched roofs and adobe walls, ideal hiding places for these bugs. In such situations they can be killed by means of blow-lamps and similar appliances which scorch their retreats and insecticides can be sprayed into these. Their control is, however, all the more difficult because they maintain themselves on many kinds of wild animals as well as upon man.

WHY WORRY ABOUT PARASITIC ANIMALS?

THE preceding chapters of this book will have given the reader some idea of the different types of injury inflicted on man by parasitic animals, but they have not discussed the total sum of economic losses, suffering and mortality that the diseases caused by parasitic animals inflict on human civilization. A few words on this subject may succeed in indicating, in the brief space available, that all the effort expended by the governments of all progressive countries in the world on the control of parasitic animals and all the vast sums of money expended on the battle against these scourges, are absolutely necessary. Parasitic animals not only cause, in man and other animals, incalculable suffering and kill great numbers of people, but they may also, if they are not controlled, make it impossible for man to live in certain parts of the world. They can seriously disrupt man's industrial organizations and they inflict on his domesticated animals, upon which man depends for his supplies of meat, milk, eggs, and other important foods, losses the extent of which is rarely fully realized.

If we look first into the direct effects of parasitic animals on human life, we find that from earliest times man has been their victim. The mummies of Egypt show evidence of common infection of the people of the Nile Valley with a species that was probably *Schistosoma haematobium*; the old-world hookworm, *Ancylostoma duodenale*, is mentioned in the Papyrus Ebers dated 1600 B.C. and this Papyrus also described a worm that was probably the beef tapeworm, *Taenia saginata*. The Persian physician Avicenna, who lived between the years A.D. 981 and 1037 also described this worm, together with the old-world hookworm, the human threadworm, *Enterobius vermicularis*, and also *Ascaris lumbricoides*. He also knew about filariasis, caused by Bancroft's filarial worm, *Wuchereria bancrofti*. This latter disease was, however, known to the Hindus in 600 B.C. We cannot be certain that the fiery serpent mentioned in the Bible (Numbers, Chap. 21, v. 6) as a plague of the Israelites when they were crossing the Red Sea, was the Guinea worm, *Dracunculus medinensis,* but many experts consider that it was. What species are referred to in ancient Chinese documents we cannot be certain, but as Craig and Faust (1955) remark, ancient Chinese folklore states that the God of creation brushed the lice off his body and created man from them. Nor can we have any accurate conception of the numbers of people who were infected by parasitic animals in these early times, but the incidence of them in man was probably much higher then, because so little was known about them. Little has been known, in fact, throughout most of the history of man. Only quite recently did we begin to acquire the extensive knowledge of them that we now have.

An impetus to the study of their life histories and biology was given by the invention of the microscope and by the brilliant use made of primitive forms of it by Van Leeuwenhoek (1632–1723) and others who followed him. The improvements in the microscope that came later, made it possible to study the microscopic phases of parasitic animals, but no appreciable advance was made till a century later, when, in the 1850's, the life histories of the pork tapeworm, *Taenia solium* and the hydatid tapeworm, *Echinococcus granulosus,* were worked out. After Manson's discovery, in 1878–9, that Bancroft's filarial worm is transmitted to man by mosquitoes, the details of the life histories of the malarial parasites of birds and man and of those of other species were worked out. Another of the earliest life histories to be worked out was the life history of the liver fluke of sheep and cattle, *Fasciola hepatica.* The adult fluke had been discovered by the French shepherd, Jean de Brie, in 1379; but it was not until 1883 that Thomas in England and Leuckart in Germany independently worked out its life history. The greater part of our knowledge of parasitic animals of all kinds has therefore been acquired during the lives of octogenarian people nowadays alive, so that it is not surprising that we know little of the actual numbers of parasitic animals that infected our ancestors.

We know, however, a great deal more about their prevalence today. Stoll (1947), for example, estimated that there were in the world at the time when he made his calculations enough infestations with parasitic worms of various kinds to provide one infection for almost every person in the world; and he made also estimates of the numbers of people infected with various species of these worms and gave, as acccurately as he could, the geographical distribution of each species. Some of his estimates have been quoted earlier in this book and they need not be repeated here. The World Health Organization (1955) states that some 250 million people in the world nowadays have clinical attacks of malaria each year and that this disease kills some $2\frac{1}{2}$ millions of people every year. Possibly these estimates understate the incidence of these parasites, because information about their incidence and effects in Russia and China is not so full as it is from other countries. Malaria is, as chapter 8 explains, being rapidly controlled in many countries and from some it has been virtually or completely eradicated, largely by the use of the new insecticides. Trypanosomiasis is also no longer a major scourge in parts of Africa, although constant vigilance is necessary to make sure that it does not evade the methods of control used against it. In South America control of the form of it that occurs there is more difficult. Amoebic dysentery is, we now know, a disease caused by an amoeba that lives as a harmless commensal in many people, but may become, under certain circumstances, a parasite that causes disease. As soon as we understand what factors cause it to do this, the control or eradication of this disease will be more effective.

Much more could be written about the direct effects of parasitic animals on human life and health, but enough has been said to show that they cause incalculable suffering and the loss of many lives. How else do they affect man? Put into a single sentence, their other effects are to make difficult, or impossible, the colonization of certain areas in the world, especially some parts of the tropics, to cause so much ill-health and consequent inefficiency that industry and other human activities are handicapped, and to inflict enormous losses on the animals upon which man relies for his supplies of meat, milk and eggs.

Animals Parasitic in Man

To a world in which human beings are becoming so numerous that man is seriously concerned lest there may not be in the future sufficient supplies of human food, any cause of serious losses of domesticated animals must be an important consideration. Do parasitic animals kill off many of these essential sources of food? There is plenty of evidence that, in spite of all our efforts to prevent them doing this, they are a serious menace to our food supplies in every country in the world.

It is always difficult to assess with accuracy the extent of losses caused by disease, whatever its cause, of domesticated animals. Some attempts to do this have, however, been made. One of the most careful of them was carried out by the United States Bureau of Animal Industry (1942). This estimate stated the annual losses in financial terms. It put the total losses caused by diseases of domesticated animals caused by bacteria, viruses and parasitic animals at 418 million dollars a year and estimated that about 69 per cent of this total loss, that is to say, about 292 million dollars a year, must be ascribed to parasitic animals of various kinds. Dr Hagan (1947), a distinguished American veterinarian, placed the total figure at 1,000 million dollars a year at least. According to *Veterinary Medicine* (1956) losses in the United States due to parasites alone are nowadays approaching this figure. Losses due to the deaths of domesticated animals are not the only ones that disease inflicts. Diseases also retard the growth of these animals and diminish their output of such foods as milk and eggs and they may injure their breeding capacity, so that their effects extend beyond the individuals of any particular generation. Sick animals also require care and they need additional foods, the consumption of which may decrease the food supplies of healthy stock. These further sources of loss must therefore be added to our estimates of the total losses incurred. Diseases caused by some kinds of parasitic animals, such as the roundworms parasitic in the food canal and lungs and the protozoan trypanosomes and the coccidia which cause coccidiosis of poultry, undoubtedly cause a great deal of harm of this kind. They cause deaths; but they also cause a great deal of unthriftiness and diminished productivity as well. No-one acquainted with the facts would deny that 'poor doing', as the farmer graphically expresses these states of chronic ill-health, is the cause of a great deal of loss of the products of domesticated animals.

The estimate given above applies, of course, only to the United States. The United States, it may be argued, is a big country that carries a great number of domesticated animals of all kinds, so that the figures just quoted may give a distorted impression of the magnitude of the losses inflicted. Any estimate of this kind must, of course, be approximate and it must be related to the number of domesticated animals carried by the country in which it is made. More important still, it must also be related to the standards of care and veterinary supervision provided by that country. In the United States these standards are high, much higher than those of many other countries. We can therefore expect to find, in other less highly organized countries, a higher rather than a lower loss from causes of this kind.

We are, moreover, estimating here only the losses inflicted by parasitic animals on our animal sources of food. If we add to these the enormous damage inflicted on our food crops, the total losses inflicted by parasitic animals of all kinds on the food supplies of the world become, indeed a menace of the first magnitude.

There is not space in this book to discuss at any length the effects of parasitic animals in preventing, or making difficult, the colonization of certain parts of the world. The description given in chapter 8 of the effects that malaria may have convinced the reader that this disease, at any rate, may make it difficult for human communities to exist in areas in which it is prevalent. Trypanosomiasis may have the same effect in Africa; its effects are all the greater because of the fact that it attacks, not only man, but also the cattle and other domesticated animals on which man depends; and in chapter 9 it was explained that the removal of whole human settlements has been necessary in parts of Africa. To describe in any detail the effects that some parasitic animals may have on human industries and other occupations would require a great deal more space than is available here. We must be content to point out that the species of parasitic animals that do not kill men, women and children, but cause in them instead such debilitating diseases as anaemia, inevitably reduce the efficiency of populations stricken by them, causing not only physical weakness, but also mental dullness and inertia. When, as so often happens, malnutrition, overcrowding, and bad housing and sanitation add their effects to those of the effects of the parasitic animals, the results are accentuated. This is the picture created by such parasitic animals as the hookworms, which can remove remarkable amounts of blood from man. American and Japanese workers who watched the dog hookworms. *Ancylostoma caninum* actually sucking blood from the small intestine of a living, anaesthetized dog, calculated that each hookworm could remove at least 0·5 c.c. of blood a day; 500 of these hookworms could therefore remove 250 c.c. (nearly half a pint) of blood. If we include also the blood lost from bleeding sites abandoned by the hookworms, which go on bleeding because the worms have injected substances (*anticoagulins*) into them which prevent the clotting of the blood, the total loss of blood is greater than this. We are not, perhaps, entitled to assume that the human hookworms suck blood at the same rate as this, and it does not follow that hookworms of any species go on sucking blood at this rate all the time; but the facts just stated explain how it comes about that the hookworms cause severe anaemia. American workers have estimated that about 500 human hookworms are required to produce a condition of disease in a healthy adult human being who is taking adequate amounts of the iron needed for the manufacture of the haemoglobin of the blood. In poorly-nourished individuals even 25 hookworms may cause anaemia. In children 100 hookworms may cause disease; and pregnant women whose iron is being depleted by the needs of the children in their wombs may be severely affected. The anaemia can, however, usually be overcome by the administration of iron and eliminated by the removal of the worms.

This interlude on blood-sucking, unpleasant reading though it may be, does show us how a parasitic animal may cause, not so much the death of the people it infects, but continued debility and inefficiency, which, if they affect whole populations, have serious social and economic effects. Among children especially effects of this kind may be severe and very sad. Their growth is stunted, their mental development is retarded and apathy and inaction replace the vigour and intelligence that should be theirs by right.

Hookworms, of course, are not alone in inflicting sufferings of this kind on the human race. Most of the other species described in this book can inflict similar sufferings and similar loss of efficiency and social effects. The horrible deformities and other effects caused by such species as the leishmanias, the blood-flukes, and the filarial roundworms must be seen if their full effects on the individuals who suffer them are to be fully realized. The fullest realization of their total effects comes, perhaps, only to the doctors, biologists, research workers, and others of every nationality, who strive, often at the risk of acquiring fatal diseases themselves, and sometimes at the cost of their own lives, to banish these scourges of human life from the world. The devotion and self-sacrifice of these workers, and the equal devotion and self-sacrifice of all the people who help them in various capacities, does not receive the attention and gratitude that it so richly deserves. It is, in a world distracted by personal and national fears and never for long relieved of the threat of wars, famines, and other calamities, a proof that there still exist a great many people who, whatever the consequences to themselves may be, concentrate their energies and thoughts on the sufferings of their fellow human beings and, thinking and acting objectively, put into hard and exacting practice that basic principle of self-denial which is among the highest achievements of civilized man. If this book, small as it necessarily is, can draw attention to this fact, it will have realized one of its several purposes.

Further Reading

(Most of the literature about the parasitic animals that are described in this book is written for medical men or parasitologists, but it is given in the following list either because it is quoted in this book or because some readers may wish to consult it. All the books or articles mentioned in this list contain further references to the extensive literature of parasitology. The items which the general reader will find most interesting are marked with an asterisk.)

Allen, G. M. *1940. *Bats*. Harvard University Press, Cambridge, Mass. (2nd Edn. 1962, Dover Publications, N.Y.)

Baker, E. W., and Wharton, G. W. 1952. *An Introduction to Acarology*. The Macmillan Co., New York.

Balfour, A., and Scott, H. H. 1924. 'Health Problems of the Empire.' Quoted by Sinton, J. A. 1935. *Rec. Malar. Survey, India*, **5**, 428.

Belding, D. L. 1952. *Textbook of Clinical Parasitology*, D. Appleton-Century-Crofts, New York.

Blacklock, D. B., and Southwell, T. 1953. *A Guide to Human Parasitology*, revised by Davey, T. H. H. K. Lewis, London.

Boyd, M. F. 1949. *Malariology*. Vols I and II, with articles by 69 experts. W. G. Saunders, Philadelphia and London.

Brumpt, E. 1949. *Précis de Parasitologie*. Masson, Paris.

Buchsbaum, R. *1938. *Animals without Backbones*. University of Chicago Press, Illinois, U.S.A. and Cambridge University Press, London.

1951. Issued as a Pelican Book, Penguin Books, Harmondsworth, Middlesex.

Buxton, P. A. 1939. *The Louse*. Arnold, London.

*1948. *Trypanosomiasis in East Africa*. H. M. Stationery Office, London.

1955. *The Biology of the Tsetse Flies*. Memoir No. 10. London School of Hygiene and Tropical Medicine. H. K. Lewis. London.

Caullery, M. *1952. *Parasitism and Symbiosis*, (translated from the French by Dr Averil M. Lysaght). Sidgwick and Jackson, London.

Chandler, A. C. *1955. *Introduction to Parasitology*. John Wiley, and Sons, New York and Chapman and Hall, London. (10th Edn. 1961, by Clark P. Read and the late A. C. Chandler.)

Further Reading

Covell, Sir G., *et al.* 1955. *The Chemotherapy of Malaria.* World Health Organization, Monograph Series, No. 27.

Craig, C. F., and Faust, E. C. 1955. *Clinical Parasitology.* Henry Kimpton, London. (6th Edn. 1957, by Faust, E. C., Russell, P. F., and Lincicome, D. R.)

Davey, T. H. *1948. *Trypanosomiasis in British West Africa.* H. M. Stationery Office, London.

Dawes, B. 1946. *The Trematoda.* Cambridge University Press, Cambridge and London.

Elton, C. 1933. *The Ecology of Animals.* Methuen, London.

Fairley, Sir H. *1947. 'The Fight against Disease.' *Journal of the Research Defence Society*, **35**, 2–19.

Ferris, G. F. 1951. *The sucking Lice, Vol. I. Memoirs of the Pacific Coast Entomological Society*, California Academy of Sciences, San Francisco, 18.

Graham-Smith, G. S. 1913. *Flies in Relation to Disease. Non-bloodsucking Flies.* Cambridge University Press, Cambridge and London.

Hagan, W. A. 1947. *Annals New York Academy of Sciences.* **48**, 351.

Hoare, C. A. 1949. *Handbook of Medical Protozoology.* Baillière, Tindall and Cox, London.

Howard, L. O. 1909. *Bull. U.S. Bureau Entomology*, No. 78.

Imms, A. D. 1934. *A General Textbook of Entomology.* Methuen, London. (9th Edn. revised by Richardson, O. W., and Davies, R. G.)

Kudo, R. R. 1954. *Protozoology.* C. C. Thomas, Springfield, Illinois, U.S.A.

Lapage, G. *1948. 'Parasitic Animals and the World's Food.' *Endeavour*, **7**, 27.

*1950. 'Parasites and War.' *Endeavour*, **9**, 134.

*1951. *Parasitic Animals.* Cambridge University Press, Cambridge and London. (2nd Edn. 1958, Heffer, Cambridge.)

*1952. 'The Battle with the Trypanosomes.' *Discovery*, **13**, 224 and 256.

1956. *Veterinary Parasitology.* Oliver and Boyd, Edinburgh and London.

1956. *Mönnig's Veterinary Helminthology and Entomology*, 4th Edition, Baillière, Tindall and Cox, London. (5th Edn. 1962.)

Manson-Bahr, Sir P. H. 1954. *Manson's Tropical Diseases.* Cassell, London. (15th Edn. 1961.)

*McNalty, Sir A. 1943. 'Indigenous Malaria in England.' *Nature*. April 17, 440.

Matheson, R. 1950. *Medical Entomology*. Comstock Publishing Co., New York and Constable, London.

*Mellanby, K. 1943. *Scabies*. Oxford University Press, London.

*Moreton, B. D. 1952. *A Guide to British Insects*. Macmillan, London.

Morgan, B. B., and Hawkins, P. A. 1948. *Veterinary Protozoology*. Burgess Publishing Co., Minneapolis, U.S.A.

Palmer, 1955. *American Journal of Tropical Medicine*, **4**, 756–7.

Pillers, A. W. N. 1921. *Notes on Mange and Allied Mites*. Baillière, Tindall, and Cox, London.

*Rothschild, M., and Clay, T. 1952. *Fleas, Flukes and Cuckoos*. Collins, London.

Sinton, J. A. 1935. *Rec. Malar. Survey, India*, **5**, 427.

Smart, J. 1948. *Handbook for the Identification of Insects of Medical Importance*. Trustees of the British Museum, London.

*Soper, F. L., and Wilson, D. B. 1943. *Anopheles gambiae in Brazil, 1930 to 1940*. The Rockefeller Foundation, New York.

Smit, F. G. A. M. 1952. *Bulletin of the World Health Organization*, v. **7**, 323.

1954. *Handbook for the Identification of British Insects*, I, No. 16. Royal Entomological Society, London.

Stoll, N. R. 1947. 'This Wormy World.' *Journal of Parasitology*, **43**, p. 1.

Thornton, H. 1952. *A Textbook of Meat Inspection*. Baillière, Tindall and Cox, London.

U.S. Bureau of Animal Industry, *Year Book of the U.S. Department of Agriculture*, 1942. U.S. Govt. Printing Office.

Veterinary Medicine, 1956, v. **57**, p. 573.

Wardle, R. A., and McLeod, J. A. 1952. *The Zoology of the Tapeworms*. University of Minnesota Press, Minneapolis, U.S.A.

Williams, L. L. 1938. 'New Jersey Mosquito Extermination Association,' quoted in Boyd, *Malariology*.

*World Health Organization, *Chronicle*, 1955, v. **9**, p. 31. *Ibid.* 1956, v. **10**, p. 354; 1961, v. **16**, 9; and *passim*.

Index

Aberrant parasites, 21, 58
Abnormal host, 37
Abortion of cattle, 210
Acanthocephala, 258
Acanthocheilonema perstans, see *Dipetalonema perstans*
Acaricides, 278, 295
Acarina, 241
Accidental parasites, 21
Acquired immunity to parasitic animals, 275–7
Aedes, 98, 106, 159
Aeroplanes, spraying of insecticides by, 296
Algerian Dragon, 212
Alternation of generations, 267
Alternative hosts, 36
Amblyomma, transmission of diseases by, 246
American Mountain fever, 246
American murderer, 41
American screw-worm fly, 236
Amoeba proteus, 24
Amoebic dysentery, 48, 49; control, 281; see also *Entamoeba histolytica*
Amphibia, 186
Anal strut, 224, 225
Ancylostoma, braziliense, hosts and geographical distribution, 41; causing creeping eruption, 44; *caninum*, hosts and geographical distribution, 41; amount of blood removed by, 302; *ceylanicum*, hosts and geographical distribution, 41; *duodenale*, anatomy, host, and geographical distribution, 39–41; causing ground-itch, 44; control, 290–1; effects on man, 301–2; egg-production, 261–2; life history, 29, 30; longevity, 261; world incidence in man, 42
Ancylostomiasis, 301–2
Ancylostomatidae, 40
Animal associations, 14–16
Annelida, 25, 39, 211

Anopheles, 99, 100, 106, 159; method of sucking blood, 178; *darlingi*, 176; *funestus*, 176; *gambiae*, 165, 166, 176; *maculipennis*, 177,178; *maculipennis* var. *atroparvus*, 176; *minimus*, 176; *punctulatus*, 176; *stephensi*, 176; *sundaicus*, 176; *superpictus*, 176
Antenna, 27; of flea, 223
Antennal groove, 223
Anthrax, 234
Anthelmintics, 278
Antibodies, 274–5
Anticoagulins, 40, 212, 302
Antimalarial drugs, 181–2, 278
Aphids, 232
Apple-sucker, 232
Arachnida, parasitic in man, 27, 241–53; egg-production, 263–4; mouth parts, 218–20
Argasidae, 242
Armillifer, armillatus, 252; *moniliformis*, 252
Arthropoda, characters and classification, 26–8; control of blood-sucking species, 293–6
Artificial immunity, 275–6
Ascaris lumbricoides; aberrant in larvae of, 58; anatomy, hosts, effects on the hosts, and life history, 57–63; causing intestinal obstruction, 58, Plate 4a; control, 280–1; dispersal of the eggs of, 280–1; egg-production, 63, 261; longevity, 62; migration of the larvae, 61–2; physiological strains, 57; resistance of the eggs, 60–1; world incidence in man, 58
Assassin bug, 201, 232; see also Reduviidae
Associations, animal, 14–16
Attachment to the host, modes of, 255–7
Auchmeromyia luteola, habits, hosts, and effects on the hosts, 236–7
Australorbis, 94

307

Index